TH

PERFUMES

JOHN OAKES

HarperCollins*Publishers*

HarperCollins*Publishers*

First published in Australia in 1996

HarperCollins*Publishers*
25 Ryde Road, Pymble, Sydney NSW 2073, Australia
31 View Road, Glenfield, Auckland 10, New Zealand
77–85 Fulham Palace Road, London W6 8JB, United Kingdom
Hazelton Lanes, 55 Avenue Road, Suite 2900, Toronto, Ontario, M5R 3L2
and 1995 Markham Road, Scarborough, Ontario, M1B 5M8, Canada
10 East 53rd Street, New York NY 10032, United States of America

National Library of Australia Cataloguing-in-Publication data:

Oakes, John.
The book of perfumes.
Includes index
ISBN 0 7322 5705 0.

1. Perfumes – History. I. Title.

391.63

Cover design by Darian Causby.
Illustrations by Lynda Taylor.

Printed in Australia by Southbank Book

9 8 7 6 5 4 3 2 1
99 98 97 96

391.63
Oa
C.1   1. Perfumes–History

CONTENTS

This book is dedicated to
the woman who knows she is not
complete without the aura
of a beautiful perfume –
the one that is absolutely right for
her look, her mood, her message.

I would like to acknowledge many facts and inspirations
from *The Book of Perfume* by Elisabeth Barillé and
Catherine Laroze, published by Flammarion, and
The Fragrance Directory by Michael Edwards & Co.
Thanks also to Julia's Perfumery of Sydney for kind
assistance in sketching for the illustrations in this book,
and to the various ladies who sell perfumes in David Jones,
Elizabeth Street, for their unfailing help and enthusisam.

MY
PERFUMED
PAST

An introduction

*H*ow did I come to write this little book? Where did my love of perfume come from? And how do I know what I'm talking about in what is presumed to be a strictly female domain?

I have always been fascinated by pleasant smells – from food, from nature, from other people, but mostly from beautiful bottles with impossible names in impossibly beautiful boxes.

Born in the tropics, in Far North Queensland, from childhood I was surrounded with the powerful smells of luscious fruits, salty winds and even saltier seas, and a plethora of highly fragrant flowers, grasses, vines and trees. Virtually at the end of our backyard loomed Queensland's highest mountain, Bartle Frere, where a great uncle climbed by night to collect orchids nobody else in the world had seen. My grandmother had an enormous garden full of wild and wonderful things. The entire family made wondrously exotic chutneys, jams, pickles and preserves from the fruits and vegetables that literally fell into our laps. I was free to wander through lush rainforests long before they were endangered and polluted, so I came to smell all the various emanations from the moist earth and the dripping vegetation first-hand. I was so naturally immersed in this highly scented, voluptuous world, I thought it was the norm!

It came as something of a surprise, then, to have a mother who appreciated all things beautiful except what she called 'scent'. She didn't dislike it; she said she simply didn't need it. My aunts were made of less stern stuff, and I began to realise they doted on it. One in particular mortally offended my mother by appearing at a ladylike afternoon tea party drenched in the latest sensation, a perfume called **Apple Blossom**, which was made by the formidable Helena Rubinstein. **Apple Blossom**, especially in very warm tropical conditions, was not what you'd call subtle. It pervaded the room, completely eclipsing the gently dabbed **No. 4711 Eau de Cologne** and Yardley **Lavender Water** wafting discreetly from the lace and lawn hankies of the other ladies. My mother even accused it of ruining her best passionfruit sponge with its overpowering 'pong', as she impolitely termed it, and was glad to see the back of the offending aunt. I, of course, loved it!

This aunt, who was considered rather *risqué*, living as she did in the Big Smoke of Brisbane and holding down a job in a department store, promoted **Apple Blossom** in the most tactile way of all – by wearing it in various forms (soap, talc, perfume, bubble bath, bath oil) in the most lavish quantities. She was actually an unwitting forerunner of the technique women now know as 'layering a fragrance'.

My first interest in commercially available perfumes was largely due to my aunt. She promoted the entire Rubinstein range (which then consisted of such lovelies as **White Magnolia**, **Heaven Sent** – or was it **Heaven Scent**? – and **Noa-Noa**, which was often called 'Krakatoa' by its detractors). It all made me curious about the power of perfume and how it could arouse passion, awaken memories and provoke a fierce sense of self-identification.

In my early teens I was sent to school in Brisbane and lived with my Apple-Blossomed aunt who, it turned out, also had a stockpile of rarely worn French perfumes, courtesy of various gentleman callers, I think. I was discreet enough not to ask how she acquired them, but the very sight of them in their bottles brought her to a romantic flood of tears. Maybe she associated them with some grand passion of the past? She did at last let me have a whiff of them, and from that moment on, **Apple Blossom** bit the dust. I learned quickly: if it was perfume, it had to be French! Soon the time came when I was old and brave enough to lurk around perfume counters like Coty. In those days, Coty was a highly revered name in beauty and perfumery. I doubt if I fully appreciated then the inventive, innovative genius and showmanship of François Coty, and I am bitterly disappointed that his name now means little in the world of perfume.

I discovered that Coty's great perfumes – **L'Aimant** (still miraculously available), **Paris** (long before YSL), **L'Origan**, **Rose Jacqueminot**, **Nouveau Gardénia**, **Muguet des Bois**, **Emeraude** and the 'green' that once changed the entire course of perfumery, the great **Chypre** – were all available as hair brilliantines! That was my opening – the legitimate and unembarrassing way I could try these magical smells. It was as if the gates of heaven had opened for me.

The step from Coty to Caron, to Guerlain, Schiaparelli and the rest was a natural one. I had passed the window of a Ladies' Beauty and Hairdressing Salon a few times on the way home from high school, and was mesmerised by the extraordinary display of glittering, glamorous-looking perfume bottles arrayed in all their Gallic splendour. A little gypsy-like lady inside spied me and came to the door to ask if I'd like some help. Well! She helped me to a feast of dazzling delights, perfumes which were to establish my insatiable thirst for knowledge of all things perfumed. She gave me, through her own knowledge and guidance, a priceless legacy that has never ceased to absorb and fascinate me.

Of course, like Marcel Proust had discovered, a lot of the things I once treasured have been forgotten over the years, and it never ceases to amaze and annoy me that some of the world's most glorious and unique perfumes have disappeared altogether – or at least from the ruthlessly pruned stocklists of perfume distributors. Worst of all, no other perfumes seem to have adequately replaced them. But, in hindsight, they are the ones that taught me the most – about finesse, about fearlessness, about difference!

People are always asking me what my favourite perfume is. I can answer that easily, but not without a little regret, because it's no longer available – at least not in its original form. From the moment I first sniffed it, **Vent Vert** by Pierre Balmain has been my all-time favourite. This is the quintessential 'green' beauty, invented in 1947 by Germaine Cellier, one of the few great female 'noses'. It still sends a shiver down my spine with its sharply evocative smell of new-mown grass, its subtle hints of windblown cinnamon and nutmeg and its raunchy fresh herbs and wild tangles of flowers. That's the original. The revamped version is much the same, only more powdery and less demonstrative, but at least it's still basically **Vent Vert**, so all is not lost! It had a distant relative by Carven called **Vert et Blanc** (which was created for Grace Kelly's wedding to Prince Rainier). This was even sharper and more astringent – too much so for the timid, but not for me!

But it had some pretty stiff competition in favouritism. Those of us who remember the wild orientalism of Lancôme's **Sikkim** will wonder why it disappeared without warning, closing the very gates of Shangri-la in our disappointed faces. Likewise the bravest and most uncompromising oriental of all time, Caron's **Poivre** (literally 'pepper'), that could cut a swathe through a room like a devastating scimitar; also by Caron, the wildly beautiful **Les Pois de Senteur de Chez Moi** ('The Sweetpeas at My Place'), perhaps still available in Paris. This perfume didn't smell just like sweet sweetpeas but like a whole trellis of them running rampant – leaves and all!

Then there was the dark green elegance of Raphael's **Réplique** – a rich and haughty empress that smelled like liquid emeralds; and the two renegades from Christian Dior – the sparkling, zany, effervescent zip and zap of **Dior-Dior** and the uncompromising drama of **Diorama**, which always guaranteed a grand entrance. Both these perfumes are sorely missed for their arrogant, unconventional attitudes. Also unforgettable is the elegantly enigmatic oriental green sophistication of Millot's classic **Crêpe de**

Chine. Then there was the almost vulgar but typically roaring twenties' fun of Dana's two party girls, **20 Carats** (it had flecks of gold floating in its Art Deco bottle) and its sister **Platine** (which featured silver flecks, of course). Still available at boutiques is the fabulous creamy artistry of Pierre Balmain's **Ivoire**, which always reminds me of the scent of my grandmother's garden after a shower of rain; and the enchantingly young and virginal **Casaque** by Jean D'Albret, a perfume that is all trembling delicacy laden with innocent nostalgia.

My love affair with perfume has not been too seriously injured by the disappearance of these favourites. If anything, it's been intensified. Perfumes evolve all the time in endless variations on classic themes or totally new and daring ideas, so why resist them? To me, perfume is a never-ending fascination, and I hope that through this book I can pass on a sense of discovery, adventure and love for one of the world's most pleasurable creations.

The adventure begins

This book sets out to tell you how to be beautifully fragrant. It is meant to be a simple, informative and entertaining guide to as many commercially available perfumes as space permits – what each one is like, its character, its ingredients, and its effect on the wearer and those she encounters.

It will guide you through the perils of actually choosing and buying a perfume new to you – and how to avoid confusion, indecision and mistakes before you make your choice. It also gives you a colloquial guide to the pronunciations of perfumes and their makers, so you can avoid embarrassing moments trying to get your tongue around some strange-sounding names. I've made these as simple as possible, but don't feel you're a failure if you don't sound like the real thing. Near enough is good enough.

This book doesn't delve into the whys and wherefores of perfumes or their chemical make-ups. Nor does it examine the vexing question of why certain perfumes will or will not suit you – the type of skin you have and your own personal preferences are vital factors that only you can deal with. (Incidentally, I don't often subscribe to those two chestnuts: 'I'm allergic to perfume' or 'perfume gives me a headache'. Most times it's either a silly myth or the perfume you've been wearing doesn't agree with your skin or your nose at the time. If you are truly allergic to fragrance, though, you have my deepest sympathy.)

Finally, to clarify terminology, I have opted for the word 'perfume' over 'fragrance' for the simple reason that 'fragrance' can mean something different in its own right and can be used to describe other things that eventually become the finished product – which is the 'perfume'.

So, here we go!

THE
MYSTIQUE
DEMYSTIFIED

The five perfume categories

*B*arely anything that has an odour, be it pleasant, disturbing, glorious, exotic or even downright challenging, has escaped the perfumer's nose. And that includes scents that aren't necessarily natural but have been invented in the laboratory, all in the name of perfume.

A lot of this precious gathering remains a mystery to us, but supersensitive and creative perfumers ferret out every fragrant possibility, in endless combinations, to come up with something new that might persuade our noses. These perfumers have a veritable Garden of Eden from which to choose and combine a fantastic array of scents, which is why the choices of perfumes are so bewildering. But the perfumers tend not to be overly communicative about their creations, so to make things easier for us, analysts have invaded their territory to come up with a few clues about the 'type' of perfume we might be smelling.

Flowers, of course, are the obvious ingredients on which to construct a perfume. But so, for instance, are trees – their fruits, blossoms, leaves, barks and even roots. Grasses, ferns, mosses, herbs and spices are also grist to the perfumer's mill. How they are placed – side by side, one on top of the other, marshalled up-front or in the background – and in what concentrations, is the real mystique of a perfume.

These, then, are the basic guides, the easily recognised categories or scent types you'll come across. Be aware, though, that lots of cross-pollination goes on, so that a perfume can transcend one type and cross over into another one quite smoothly.

The art of the single flower

In the latter half of the nineteenth century and the first quarter of this one, uncomplicated one-flower scents were the ones most readily available to the perfumer, as floral blends were only just becoming possible with new methods of extraction and fixing. Most of these single-flower perfumes were instantly recognisable. Indeed, a woman could become known for her fidelity to one floral scent, which more or less became her personal motif. The flowers used were the obvious choices of rose, carnation, lily, violet, lavender, lilac and gardenia.

Today these perfumes are something of a rarity, their appeal much diminished with the availability of far more complex blends. (Chanel always insisted that women didn't want to smell like a bed of roses, which led to her creation of the inextinguishable **No. 5**.) However, there is still considerable appeal in the accuracy and nostalgic charm of this category, and many perfumers have resurrected the genre with updated variations. There are some very notable examples, including the Perfumer's Workshop's **Tea Rose**, Yardley's **Lavender Water**, **Lily of the Valley**, **Roses** and **April Violets**, and Annick Goutal's **Tubereuse**, a flower which is also the dominating factor in Lagerfeld's **Chloé**. Caron dedicated **Muguet du Bonheur** to the delicate lily of the valley, as did Dior in **Diorissimo**, and Cacharel used all sorts of lilies in **Anaïs Anaïs**. Roses, in all their old-fashioned glory, are the basis of Saint Laurent's **Paris**, and Caron has been responsible for a swag of beauties inspired by the sweet pea (**Pois de Senteur**), narcissus (**Narcisse Noir**) and carnation (**Bellodgia**). So, if you don't necessarily agree with Madame Chanel's stern edict, there are still many beautiful examples of this category for the choosing and wearing, and with new techniques of extraction and the invention of hundreds of smell-alike chemical discoveries, I wouldn't be surprised at a comeback!

The floral bouquet maze

This is a veritable scented minefield when it comes to definitions. A vast number of perfumes are composed of flower essences, forming what is termed a floral bouquet. There are so many of them and some so similar in construction you may be forgiven for thinking quite a few have copied one another. But the fact is, no matter how closely one perfume resembles another, no two are exactly alike, not even technically. Which is why this category is not only the largest but also the most confusing.

The vast majority of floral perfumes are based on the tried-and-true alliance of roses and jasmine. It's a magnificent marriage and provides the romantic and persuasive basis on which all sorts of other perfume ideas can be laid. The variations on the theme are deliciously endless.

To explain what I'm talking about, let's take a couple of examples. Jean Patou's world-famous **Joy**, although the quintessential mating of Bulgarian roses and Grasse jasmine in enormously extravagant concentrations, also incorporates a reputed one hundred other essences to prop up and intensify the basic accord, to make it 'sing'. On the other hand, Lanvin's classic **Arpège** begins with the same two flowers in high concentrations but overlays them with distinct notes of lily of the valley, honeysuckle, hyacinth and lilac (as well as a powerful note of green vetyver and woody sandalwood). The result couldn't be more unlike **Joy** if it tried!

Of course, not all floral bouquets contain roses and jasmine. Many take an altogether different route by combining other flowers, such as Amazone lily with tuberose and narcissus in Elizabeth Taylor's **White Diamonds**. Not a rosebud or a jasmine sprig in sight! Yet this is almost everyone's favourite perfume category, and it's very well catered for. So, if you're allergic to roses (God help you!), then there's more than one perfume out there to come to your rescue. In the case of this category, it's very much a matter of *vive la différence*!

The greening of you

Wearing one of the so-called 'green' family is like leaping back into childhood days full of the fresh, innocent scents of fields and forests, flowerbeds and orchard groves, new-mown lawns and the entire litany of spring and summer goodies. You suddenly smell freshly cut grass after rain, leaves crushed in the hand, wildflowers picked from a dewy field, even the bright smell of freshly dried sheets on a clothesline or the warm green smell of earth after rain. It's nostalgia rampant!

Most of the perfumes in this category fall into two divisions – the chypre (pronounced 'sheep') family of resins, mosses and ferns, and the purer green family of leaves, grasses and buds. And when both are combined, you get the whole gloriously verdant picture! There are three or four classic 'greens', not all of them now readily available, but worth noting as guides to newer perfumes in the category. The first green to make its mark worldwide was probably Guerlain's delicate and mysterious **Mitsouko**, which is more in the chypre category. Then along came Coty's **Chypre**, a purer, lighter version of the same theme. In 1947 Balmain shocked the world of fragrance with the greenest green of them all – **Vent Vert**, a sharp, astringent, cool and sparkling mix of leaves, grasses, flowers and spices. In between came the wonderful classic **Crêpe de Chine**, an elegant chypre type which is unfortunately very hard to find now. There were also Coty's elegant **Emeraude** and Raphael's grandly green **Réplique**, both sadly lost to us. Then, to everyone's surprise, Paloma Picasso carried on the tradition with her **Mon Parfum**, a very spicy and sophisticated green introducing a clear signal of sexiness.

Although **Vent Vert** remains the prototype, many other greens have followed, crossbreeding their greenness with multi-floral overlays and citrus notes and underlining them with dashes of herbs and spices. But no matter whether they're aligned to the countryside or to the cultivated glasshouse breed, greens are unrivalled for freshness and youthfulness. You'll recognise one the second you smell it!

Into the woods

Here you enter the darker fantasy land of pixillated smells and spells woven with imaginative whimsy and mystery. This 'woody' or 'woodsy' category is a labyrinth of smoky, earthy, ambery, foresty fragrances gathered from ferns, mosses, bark, resins, lichen, leaves, roots and timbers.

Straight-out examples of the woods family are a rarity now. The fashion for unadulterated sandalwood, cedarwood, *fougère* (fern) and so on has long since passed, and you'll find the stronger concentrations of these essences now used mostly in men's fragrances. But there are more than a few that have their roots firmly planted in the forest, notably Chanel's earthy masterpiece, **No. 19**, and Claude Montana's foresty, spicy **Montana**. The same could be said for Jean Desprez's great classic, **Bal à Versailles**, which interweaves flowers with a high concentration of sandalwood, and the darkly mysterious woods-at-night scent of Lancôme's **Magie Noire**. In fact, most of the perfumes in this neck of the woods (so to speak) are laced with multi-flowers and spices to soften the sombreness of the wood content and to intensify it with an almost hypnotic glow. But for sheer warmth and earthiness, they're unbeatable – and highly individual at that.

Fruit for all seasons

This is the luscious, almost edible category, containing perfumes so downright delicious they seem to instantly soothe the olfactory senses with the rich, ripe, mellow or sharp smells of peach, plum, apricot, berries and citrus –

even including such salivating surprises as blackcurrant, grape, mango and passionfruit. These essences are used as top notes and then underscored with compatible flowers and spices, usually with touches of greenery, and often fixed with musk and amber as a haunting counterpoint.

Some of the fruit-dominated perfumes are honey-smooth and aristocratic, like Rochas's grand classic, **Femme**. Others, such as Valentino's melon-laced **V**, are more full-throated and sunny, while Armani's glowing **Gio** and Lancôme's lemon-leaved **Ô de Lancôme** are more frankly exuberant and aggressive in a charming, captivating way.

Recently, a whole new brigade of fruity perfumes has come marching into perfume counters offering added zest and freshness. Such perfumes include Nina Ricci's **Deci Dela**, Givenchy's **Fleur d'interdit**, Cacharel's **Eden**, Clarins's **Elysium** and Calvin Klein's **Escape**, all of them ready for the plucking. You'll find the perfumes of this category not only hard to resist but a welcome change from the stranglehold of the seductive flower brigade.

Oriental persuasions

East meets west with a vengeance! The great vogue for all things oriental started after the end of World War I and dominated the twenties and early thirties with a lot of hooched-up mysticism and *femme fatale* seduction that bordered on the ridiculous. Suddenly, everything was 'forbidden' (meaning desirable) and loaded with meaningful messages. Perfumes naturally followed suit.

When the fad had had its day, most of the boudoir perfumes reeking of musk, patchouli, carnation, jasmine and roses evaporated into thin air. Chanel was the main cause of their passing with her revolutionary **No. 5**. But although most of the oriental caravan disappeared into the desert, classics like **Shalimar** and **Tabu** toughed it out with sheer class. In fact, **Shalimar** still dominates this category and is easily capable of eclipsing upstart sirens arriving on the scene.

The sixties saw a huge comeback for the orientals, both those that are pure and powerful, and multi-florals with more than a light touch of the oriental bazaar. And what a fascinating breed they are, especially the pure ones! Not for the dainty or faint-hearted, they come on strong and stay that way for a lot longer than their more refined sisters. Their compositions are usually based on the likes of patchouli, vetyver grass, musk, amber, strong herbs and even stronger spices mixed with flowers associated with the Orient – such as rose and jasmine, carnation and peony, tuberose and ylang ylang. All of this makes for an over-powering intensity, so ingredients that add softness and roundness, such as vanilla and sandalwood, are called upon to keep things on the civilised side.

These orientals naturally have a reputation as seduc-tresses, and most of them are pretty adept at shedding a few veils. They are lusty, ravishing and provocative, famous for their staying power, especially in the confines of the harem or boudoir. Just think of Saint Laurent's **Opium**, Lauder's

Cinnabar, Fendi's **Asja**, Calvin Klein's **Obsession** and Dior's **Dioressence** (not for a moment forgetting the almighty **Shalimar**) and you'll know what I mean when I say that the right woman in the right oriental perfume doesn't really give her rivals a fighting chance.

Finally, there is also a newly invented category cutely and self-consciously called 'floriental' – a generally half-hearted mixture of flowers with a faint hint of oriental spices and woods. These perfumes may appeal to the less-than-committed wearer of timid tastes.

So there you are – the basics basically described. Don't ever be frightened off by a certain category. One thing you can be pretty certain of is that within every category and its offshoots or crossbreeds, you'll find at least one perfume that will add itself quite naturally and amiably to your perfume wardrobe. After all, it's rather boring to smell continually like a flowerbed or an Indian bazaar . . . or even a field of new-mown grass!

COMING TO TERMS WITH TERMS

Ingredients

To become versed in the mysterious parlance of perfume, it is essential that you understand a few vital terms and ingredients. The short glossary of terms which follows does not claim to be a comprehensive one but rather an explanation of a few of the strange but commonly used words you will encounter in this book.

Aldehyde

PRONUNCIATION: AL-da-hide

In the early twenties Gabrielle Chanel, already a sensation of Parisian *haute couture*, decided that the House of Chanel should have its very own perfume – a new concept in those days. She prevailed upon the great perfumer Ernest Beaux to create a signature perfume for her, her only stipulation being that it had to stop the world in its tracks.

Clever Monsieur Beaux had long known about the availability of new synthetic perfume ingredients. Some of these were remarkably faithful to the original scents, others were not quite so recognisable. But among them were the fascinating new organic compounds called aldehydes. These were a motley lot, mostly created in the laboratory to give a smell that could be a substitute for a totally natural scent. Rather than dominate a perfumer's recipe, they added an extra dimension of versatility, while adding a character that could augment or intensify natural essences. They also added a powdery note, so the perfume's often sharp edges were rounded and softened to a new subtlety.

Most perfumers of the day thoroughly distrusted aldehydes, fearing they'd wreck the fidelity of the formula and give it a fake smell that would throw everything off balance. But not Monsieur Beaux. In his hands these upstart impostors became unique adjuncts imparting a new ambience to a perfume if used with imagination and care. The result was the now legendary **No. 5**.

The appropriate sensation Chanel desired was achieved. This single perfume unleashed the respectable use of aldehydes on the perfume world with such force and persuasion that from that day to this they remain integral to the creation of all perfumes.

Amber

Amber is an ingredient used in almost all perfumes that require a rich, warm softness. It is usually detectable in the base or lower notes – the ones you smell last as a perfume develops on your skin. Sometimes, though, amber is used earlier on to establish a golden aura from which the other ingredients emerge.

Amber itself is the processed resin of many species of fir trees. It possesses a smoky, smouldering, honeyed fragrance, and because of that it is very valuable, especially in the formulation of 'oriental' perfumes where it is used to counterbalance the often high-pitched and pungent notes of herbs and spices. 'Amber' is also commonly used as a generic term for any warm and oriental effect in a perfume.

Ambergris

PRONUNCIATION: AMBA-greece

Not to be confused with resinous amber, ambergris is an unpleasant but necessary component of many a perfume. A substance secreted from the stomach of the sperm whale, it is almost the ultimate fixative, giving perfume a longer life in the bottle and on the skin. Ambergris in its natural state is sometimes seen washed up on beaches as a nasty, fatty grey blob. Today it is so fearfully rare, and therefore expensive, that chemists have long since formulated their own synthetic version of it to make sure your favourite perfume doesn't evaporate into thin air when you apply it. They have also managed to make it smell almost pretty!

Bergamot

PRONUNCIATION: BERGA-mot (or BERGA-mo)

This is an oil, originally (and still occasionally) extracted from a sour little pear-shaped green orange, rather like a wild lemon. The fruit came to Italy via Turkey where it was known as the Bey's Pear. Although no one in their right mind would attempt to eat one, the fruit yields a most appealing and distinctive orange-like scented oil. It is a sharp, clean citrus smell with surprising depth and tenacity.

Guerlain used it to impress Napoleon in the formulation of an *eau de toilette*, and that gentleman took to it with a vengeance, probably to counter the musk that Jospehine wore and which he found overpowering. Bergamot is a necessary adjunct in *colognes* and *eaux de toilette*, while other perfumers utilise its emphatic and sunny aroma in their Mediterranean-inspired creations. Today, bergamot is chemically synthesised and is used in all of the fruity perfumes as well as floral-fruit bouquets, adding a citrus spike to otherwise mellow perfumes.

Castoreum

PRONUNCIATION: carst-OR-e-um

A lot of mysterious and unexpected things go into the making of a perfume, but happily castor oil isn't one of them. Which means that castoreum has nothing to do with the castor bean and its infamous oil.

However, in origin if not in fragrance, castoreum is far less attractive, coming as it does from the lymph glands of the Canadian beaver. Like musk, civet and ambergris, castoreum is used as an 'animal' note in perfume to add a lingering, rather sensual note when combined with prettier scents and essences. It also acts as a powerful fixative, preventing the bouquet of the perfume from disappearing quite so fast as it might. Actually, castoreum is so powerful that one part of it is sufficient to totally obliterate the combined efforts of forty other scents! Thus it is used extremely sparingly. And I can also report that the poor beaver is safer now because of the laboratory synthesisation of castoreum.

Civet

This is another fixative, one which has the dubious honour of being probably the most revolting smell to add its virtues to perfume.

Civet is secreted from a gland beneath the tail of the wild civet cat – not a pretty thought! It is extracted by very brave souls without harming the animal (civet cats are farmed now in places like Ethiopia) and used in the minutest quantities to blend with the more appealing ingredients and hold them together for a longer-lasting effect. It also has the other virtue of adding a haunting, earthy and sensuous note of its own that intensifies other ingredients. Nowadays, however, although the genuine article is still used in certain formulations, a perfectly satisfactory and more controllable synthetic substitute has been developed, so the poor little wild civet cat is not so relentlessly tampered with any more.

Eau de cologne, eau de toilette, eau de parfum, extrait

These are the four main forms of perfume, with *extrait* being the concentrate and the others diluted versions of it.

Personally, I think *extrait* is the most important and desirable form of a perfume. Although more expensive initially, it provides you with the true meaning and smell the perfumer intended, and in the long run is less expensive, especially when used in conjunction with other forms. An *extrait* has the power to unleash all sorts of emotions and pleasures, giving of itself in degrees so you can enjoy it in all its glory and complexity. To be slightly technical, it contains the highest percentage (20 to 30 per cent) of the concentrated essence diluted in 90 per cent proof alcohol – a pretty potent little proposition!

Eau de parfum is a relatively new form, pitched as it is between the concentrate and the toilet water strengths. It is almost as strong and almost as long-lasting as *extrait*, with a concentration of 10 to 20 per cent diluted in 90 per cent proof alcohol. Again, I think it is a wise economic proposition because of its fidelity to the original source. Because of this it has become the most popular form of perfume purchase. *Eau de parfum* usually comes in a spray form, which allows it to be used as a definite all-over aura of the basic essence.

Eau de toilette (toilet water) is more diluted again but is a very good representation of its mother perfume. It is also less expensive than *eau de parfum* and can be used lavishly to give an overall effect of the fragrance. Thus it is invaluable as a part of the perfume-layering process, or to be used when you feel like wearing something lighter in impact. It contains less than 10 per cent of the perfumed concentrate, again diluted in 90 per cent alcohol, and gives a gentler impression of the actual essence, with its top notes usually accented and the middle and base notes not quite so prominent or lasting.

Eau de cologne is an entity in itself rather than a dilution of a specific *extrait*. The most enduring and popular (and probably the best) example of a pure *cologne* is the perennial **No. 4711**. In terms of strength, the concentration of *eau de cologne* is usually around the 80 per cent mark, diluted in 85 per cent proof alcohol. If it's a true *cologne*, it will be based on citrus notes with flowers and spices in attendance.

Fixatives

Fixatives act as binding agents, giving off the base notes and the last notes of a perfume before it fades. They add the 'staying power' with varying degrees of tenacity, depending on what is used and how much (and also of what quality – natural fixatives might not always outlast synthetic ones but they will give the perfume more refinement and class). The great classic perfumes can thank their fixatives for their reputations to a large degree, which is another reason why they're so expensive but also why they last longer and smell nicer.

Civet, ambergris, musk, castoreum, sandalwood, vetyver, patchouli and oakmoss all have a low volatility, allowing them to 'cling' more and not evaporate like the highly volatile notes, which are usually used as the top or first smells of the perfume. Most fixatives could not exist alone because of their repellent characteristics, but in conjunction with other ingredients, they fuse and give a warmth and glow to the last stages of a perfume. They also stop a perfume from having a stale or sour effect at the end of its journey. It's a lack of good fixatives that make cheap perfumes smell cheap!

Jasmine

The scent of this incredibly beautiful blossom almost defies description, and writers have been known to go into ecstatic swoons trying to pin down its magic elusiveness. 'Ravishing', 'achingly sweet', 'mesmerising bliss' and even 'the essence of moonlight in the grove' are some insufficient attempts that don't quite describe the unique beauty of this wonderful flower.

Chemists these days see jasmine in a different, less sentimental light. It must drive them to distraction that they've not yet been able to totally synthesise with utter fidelity the elusive fragrance of living jasmine. They may have come thrillingly close, but not close enough to spell the end of commercial jasmine crops. It's a very expensive crop, one which has to be hand-picked first thing in the morning before the sun gets at it. Six kilograms of jasmine petals are needed to yield only about a gram of essential oil.

There are hundreds of varieties of jasmine grown in many countries for commercial perfume use, among them Italy, Egypt, India and Morocco, but it's generally agreed that the best jasmine comes from Grasse, the undisputed capital of the perfume world, located in Provençe in France. Without jasmine's heady and romantic scent we would be without 90 per cent of all perfumes. Admittedly, a large number of perfumers (who might not like to own up to it) use highly sophisticated jasmine synthetics for reasons of economy and stability, but the great ones wouldn't be caught dead making such heinous short cuts!

Leather

Most people express surprise or even horror when they learn that leather can be a powerful ingredient in perfume. Although these days it isn't used to the extent it was in the early decades of this century, in many perfumes it is making a comeback. It's a wonderful smell, so let's hope the engagement is not limited!

The fragrance itself comes from treating raw hide with birch tar and then boiling it until a woody, pungent essence redolent of fine, burnished leather is yielded. It has a haunting, smoky presence that combines surprisingly well with flowers and spices in perfumes of extreme sophistication and individuality. Probably the two most famous examples of the use of leather are in Chanel's aristocratic and quite beautiful **Cuir de Russie** (French for Russian leather), and Robert Piguet's powerful **Bandit**. It also is used quite extensively in men's fragrances.

Musk

What is known, often leeringly, as the aphrodisiac of the perfume world is actually a glandular secretion obtained from the male Tibetan musk deer. So there goes the glamour angle! Unfortunately, musk has become so inordinately popular over the decades that the understandably nervous musk deer is now in grave danger of extinction. Fortunately, however, science has come to the rescue once again, meeting the voracious demand for musk with more than adequate chemical versions of it.

Its proper use is as a powerful and efficient fixative, but musk also has the virtue of being a pervasively sensual ingredient and is added to an incredible number of perfumes. Used as it should be in small quantities, it gives perfumes a rich headiness, a hypnotic sweetness that lurks rather than lunges. On its own it smells repugnant, but when highly diluted it adds a sexiness that is not overt but seductive.

Myrrh

PRONUNCIATION: MER

Myrrh is a gum collected from scrubby little bushes in the Middle East by goats who are let loose amidst the foliage to emerge with the sticky stuff on their beards. This is then combed off by the goatherds and sold at the local markets to perfumers' buyers for a very pretty penny. No one is quite sure how one of the three wise men carried or presented his gift of myrrh to the infant Jesus, but it was probably on a stick, like incense.

Myrrh travels well, being highly aromatic and stable under pressure. It has acquired sacred connotations over the centuries – probably the reason why Caron named its myrrh-loaded perfume **Parfum Sacré**!

Nose

The most revered and highly paid people in the perfume industry are referred to as 'noses'. These experts can usually accurately identify a staggering number of ingredients in a perfume, sometimes as many as two hundred. A nose is the master perfumer; he (for it usually is a man) not only creates ideas for new perfumes but is also expected to forecast new fashions in fragrance.

The nose and his priceless appendage must also be able to deal with hundreds of different batches of ingredients every season to make sure they maintain the same intensity and same character before they are dispatched to the vats to be included in a master recipe. (If, for instance, the night-blooming jasmine of Grasse blooms earlier than usual and upsets manufacturers' schedules, he must be able to substitute jasmine from another source to compensate and maintain the delicate balance needed.) No computer yet invented can successfully replace a living, breathing, breath-taking nose with his consummate expertise and judgment.

Oakmoss

This most unremarkable substance is a species of lichen. It is dull grey-green in colour and exudes a rather heavy, oriental odour that is refined after picking. Growing quite readily in the mountains of northern Europe, it is most widely cultivated in the old Yugoslavia. The most remarkable thing about oakmoss (sometimes called *mousse en chine*) is its ability to impart to floral bouquets, green perfumes and heavy orientals a glorious velvety softness. It is also a good, inoffensive fixative. A whole host of hauntingly romantic and nostalgic perfumes would be sickly without its subtle and lingering effect.

Patchouli

Thank heavens the hippies have all grown up and desisted from their insistent use of this, the strongest ingredient in perfume! Back in the sixties they seemed to all but inject the stuff, but now that its days of overuse and ill-use are over, patchouli returns to us the way it should – diluted.

An oil extracted from the leaves and stems of the *Pogostemon cablin*, a shrub which is grown extensively all over south-eastern Asia, and especially in India, patchouli is so overpowering in its raw state that it has to be heavily diluted before use. It is not only a wonderful fixative but has a compellingly pungent, slightly musty smell. Without it, oriental perfumes as we know them wouldn't exist, nor would a lot of floral bouquet perfumes which use it as an exclamation point or as a source of depth to otherwise fragile flowers. Patchouli is a long-lasting ingredient, and once you know it, its fragrance is unmistakable. Those of us fortunate enough to remember Schiaparelli's sensational scent **Shocking** will know what I mean!

Rose

The undisputed queen of flowers is amazingly diverse. There are literally hundreds of types of roses, some perfumed, others spectacular but unfortunately scentless. The basis of most rose-dominated perfumes is the essence of *rose de mai* (*Rosa centifola*), a small, rather insignificant-looking rose that grows profusely in Grasse and produces a penetratingly sweet rose scent. There is also the Tea rose, which has a slight tannin undertone as used in a popular toilet water called **Tea Rose**. Bulgarian and Damascus roses are another thing altogether – very rich, opulent and aristocratic. The former is cultivated in Bulgaria's Valley of Roses and is considered the quintessential rose. From it comes the world's most expensive attar or oil essence – half a tonne of rose petals yields a mere gram of the precious attar. Bulgarian and Damascus roses turn up in all the big classics, such as **Joy**, **Arpège** and **Shalimar**. The very sweet and high-pitched white roses are lovingly used by Guerlain in **Jardins de Bagatelle** and Lancôme in **Trésor**, while the exotic Turkish rose is a dominating and voluptuous force in **Ungaro d'Ungaro**. In Saint Laurent's rose-drenched **Paris**, all sorts of old-fashioned roses rub shoulders with the more cultured company of the Damascus rose.

A great authority on perfume once said that the scent of the rose was one of the most aphrodisiac of odours – because of its narcotic effect, it brightened erotic thoughts aroused by the colour, form and texture of the flower. I'd put it more succinctly by saying that the fragrance of the rose is an unrivalled, sensuous and sexy knockout!

Sandalwood

This is a delicious and delicately scented wood from the Indian tree fetchingly called the Malabar white sandalwood. For centuries sandalwood has been revered as holy by the

Hindis, conveying as it does a host of mystical meanings. Widely grown throughout South-East Asia, its essence is actually distilled from woodchips, which is probably why it always reminds me of my old school pencilcase!

Almost priceless as a fixative, sandalwood also exudes an entrancingly soft and creamy fragrance. It is used in most oriental-type perfumes, and also to underline floral bouquet types with an insistent woody pulsation that counterpoints their sweetness. Most recently it has been used in very intense concentration in Guerlain's **Samsara** where, when combined with equally strong drifts of Indian jasmine, it creates a tranquil, almost mystical presence. It has also been the inspiration for Chanel's controversial perfume of yesteryear, **Bois des Iles**, which lately has reappeared reorchestrated for men as L'Égoiste.

Synthetics

Most modern perfumes call for a staggeringly high number of ingredients, and each one must be absolutely stable so as not to upset the others. This used to be a vexing problem for perfumers, but now that almost every ingredient has been, or can be synthesised, manufacturers cover possible losses by using a good proportion of them in the making of their fragrances. Whether they are superior to the real thing is a moot point, but synthetics should not be maligned as chemical fakes. Most perfumers these days consider them just as important as natural ingredients, and merrily mix them without the slightest hesitation or sense of guilt.

Tuberose

The reason for this flower's inclusion here is to help put a stop to the misconception that tuberose is a kind of rose. It certainly isn't. It is a member of the lily family, and doesn't smell remotely like a rose. Tuberose has an extraordinarily potent scent and is well known (sometimes disliked) for its pervasiveness. Yet in the hands of a master perfumer it is one of the most exquisite smells in all perfume.

You've probably seen the long stems of this creamy-pink trumpet-like flower in florists. Most of the grand romantic perfumes use it, some more emphatically than others (such as Lagerfeld's **Chloé**), but it's at its most disturbing and haunting when diffused with other beautifully scented flowers such as in Guerlain's **Jardins de Bagatelle** and Cartier's **Panthère**. The scent of tuberose is so pervasive and suggestive that, in the Italian Renaissance, young girls were forbidden to walk in gardens where it grew lest they be set upon by passionate males gone delirious with the lusty scent!

Violet

Here is yet another flower whose perfume is so familiar it scarcely needs any explanation. I include it simply to illustrate again that, in the wondrous world of perfume, things are not always as they seem!

It is the leaves that are mostly used in perfume, not the petals. This is mostly caused by the violet's notorious shyness, so the leaves are easier to gather and process. But there's also another secret to what we presume is the scent of the violet flower. Long ago, chemists used the root of the Florentine iris (which is called orris root when stored and dried) which produced a smell almost identical to real violet. Modern chemists came along and improved the process even further, commercially capturing the oil or essence from these roots to simulate violets, so now they have a choice of using this or the scent distilled from violet leaves. They can, of course, use a completely synthetic version which has a stronger, harsher smell.

Vanilla

Although it hardly needs introduction to cooks, this invaluable substance is extracted from the pods or beans of a climbing type of orchid. Much-prized by the Spaniards, who discovered it in Mexico, its aromatic possibilities soon became evident to the French (naturally), who used it in many a potion as a soft, enticing, almost aphrodisiacal ingredient. The Guerlain family latched onto it and used a synthesis of it called vanillan in some of their more voluptuous fragrances, most notably the sexy **Shalimar**.

Vanilla is soft and sweet with a creamy ambience. Too much of it is cloying, but a dash of it gives roundness and depth to oriental perfumes in no uncertain fashion. It is also an extremely tenacious scent and is quite recognisable (mainly through our food associations with it) at the base of many romantic and sensual perfumes, such as **Tocade** by Rochas.

Vetyver

You may also see this spelt 'vetiver', but it's the same wondrous smell. Known among botanists as cus-cus grass, vetyver grows wild in tropical Asia and its roots produce a fragrant oil. Used extensively in men's perfumes, its strong, acerbic scent is slightly musty but nevertheless greenly fresh and earthy. Used in women's perfumes it adds a marvellous astringent green note and gives very floral bouquets the piquancy they need to make them fascinating. It is, in fact, one of the principal base notes in classics such as Chanel's **No. 5**, Hermès's **Calèche**, and Lanvin's **Arpège**. It is also the saving grace of **Giorgio Beverly Hills** which, without its insistence, would be almost too cloying and strident.

Ylang Ylang

PRONUNCIATION: ee-LANG-ee-LANG
(say it as one word)

This strong, unique and utterly hypnotic scent turns up in masses of perfumes, especially those with an oriental bent. A tendril-like flower from the Philippine *Canagra odorata* tree, ylang ylang offers an emphatic and heady tropical note that blends brilliantly with more romantic-smelling flowers and fruits. On its own it's a bit too tenacious, so, like anything tropical, it must be handled with care and discretion. It's also magical with the green family of perfumes, underlining their sharpness with an exotic infiltration.

IN THE MOOD

You and your perfume

*L*ike you, a perfume has a distinct and unique personality. It's with this knowledge that you should begin your quest for the perfect perfume for you.

Having said this, there is not just one perfume that will mirror you completely. That's because you have various moods and emotions that can range from elation to sobriety, capriciousness to sheer coquettishness. Of course, you can also be many things at once. There's bound to be one perfume that complements every mood, emotion and occasion. Which leads me to the 'one-perfume woman' theory.

Personally, I think it's old-hat, unimaginative and bone lazy to keep wearing the same perfume year in year out. *You* might not tire of it, but you can bet those around you will! ('Here she comes again, reeking of **Joy**!' or worse still, '*She* doesn't wear that perfume, it wears *her*!') What I advocate is that you have at your fingertips a collection (an arsenal, a wardrobe . . . whatever you like!) of perfumes that will suit your moods, matching how you feel and look at the time. After all, you wear different clothes and accessories depending on the time of day and the occasion, so why shouldn't the same rules apply to the perfume you choose?

The basic rule is simply this: the perfume you choose to wear should be the ideal extension of your personality and the mood you're in. Incidentally, a perfume can also have the power to *change* your mood, so if you're in a temper or feel depressed, how nice it is to be able to select from your collection the one that will either calm you down or lift your spirits! That's the therapeutic beauty of perfume.

Ammunition

Perfume is really the ultimate weapon, so why not build up a formidable collection? It's a hefty initial financial outlay, I know, but not if you do it one at a time. If you can't afford the concentrate (*extrait*), then begin with the toilet water or a perfumed body lotion version of it. Get to know its fragrant effects intimately and build on it. Then you can begin the same process with another, and another. I would suggest at least four and not more than twelve, unless you're very fickle or an outright addict!

It's a good idea to map out your lifestyle – what sort of events you go to regularly, at what time and with whom. For instance, if you're a working girl, don't turn up at the office awash with something seductive like **Shalimar** or **Poison**. Something along the lines of **Deci Dela** or **Cristalle** is far more suitable – and fresher. If you're invited a lot to art gallery openings or concerts, don't swamp everyone around you with deep and meaningful perfumes like **SpellBound** or **Giorgio Beverly Hills**. You'll attract more attention with the likes of **Ysatis** or **Arpège**, and not upstage the occasion.

Plan on having a range of perfumes that might include a sexy oriental, a sophisticated multi-floral, a fresh green, a delicious fruity type, a single-flower perfume or simple bouquet for lighter occasions, and one that is your ultimate favourite – the one you've found that really does the trick!

Also take into consideration the time of day: mornings and lunchtimes are best dressed with a light floral or green perfume; afternoons are better suited to multi-florals or ambery, fruity scents; dusk and cocktail time is when you can start going all romantic and sensuous with heavier, more intricate perfumes, and the evening is ideal for the great classics or the newer breed of sexy, seductive heavies. But don't ever put one on top of the other unless you want to smell like a perfume counter at sale time!

If you start getting ideas from magazine advertisements or editorial articles on perfume, beware! They are usually mine-traps of misinformation and over-the-top hyperbole. How many times have you come across ads that have a stunning picture of a stunning woman with the equally stunning bottle and some catchcry along the lines of 'An explosion of love!' or ' Indulge yourself in total seduction'? Even editorials tend to be unhelpful, merely repeating verbatim the esoteric publicity handouts from the makers and distributors.

But of course the first hurdle is at the point of sale, the place where you're actually going to try on perfumes and hopefully make a decision. There are definite rules for this adventure, and I'll set them out in the next chapter so you can avoid all the perils and pitfalls with a bit of forearmed aplomb. So, before you go out into the cold, sit reflectively and make up your own mind what sort of person you are, what smells you like best, those you don't care for or dislike, where you're most likely to wear perfume and when. The perfume you choose is the one that welds with your intuition, your looks and your temperament. It is the one you should feel utterly at home with.

DECISIONS, DECISIONS!

Trying and buying

*F*or those of you who are versed in the art of buying a perfume, the following is probably old news. For the uninitiated, however, there's a lot to learn. It's a pretty daunting proposition trying to choose the right perfumes to suit your lifestyle, your personal pleasure, and your budget, but if you follow a few tried-and-true rules it shouldn't be too traumatic. In fact, it should be a treat.

It's always wise to go to an outlet where you'll find a good selection. A department store, pharmacy or specialist perfume boutique will be your best bet. The stock is likely to be more varied and the salesperson better equipped with the information you need. And you might also be lucky enough to find some rare perfumes not widely available.

When facing the perfume counter the first thing is not to be overwhelmed by the display of fabulous bottles and the avalanche of smells on offer. The second thing is not to be overwhelmed by the salesperson. Beware of she who leaps out at you with sample strips of the perfume she's pushing, flooding you with bits and pieces of promotional blurb that you mightn't be ready for. The first thing you must insist on is time – time to relax and chat and then try at your leisure. Fix the salesperson with your steeliest eye and outline what you're after. If you've never done it before, don't admit. Pretend you know *something* about the subject, and assume your most elegant coolness.

Three perfumes will be about as many as you can take in and evaluate without confusing your nose and getting the perfumes mixed up in your mind. If you're starting from scratch, ask the salesperson to suggest one fruity or green-based perfume, one oriental and one floral bouquet.

A lot of sellers will spray their samples onto paper strips. That's the current method, but I don't think it really gives you a proper idea of the perfume. After all, your skin isn't made of paper; it is highly complex and individual, and will react in its own way to different perfumes. If you're the polite type, go through with this facsimile exercise, and when she's finished, simply ask her to try each one on your skin. She'll probably squirt your wrists, and perhaps the crook of an elbow or your forearm. Don't let her spray them on herself – every perfume smells slightly different on every skin, and it's *your* skin that's of paramount importance here.

Don't rub the perfumes into your skin – this will only bruise or smudge their effect and crush the delicate notes they are ready to reveal to you. Let the perfumes settle and dry a little before you smell each one: the top notes (the ones you first smell) are very volatile and strong, but will shortly fade and give way to the middle notes at the heart of the perfume. It's the combination of these two notes that give you its message. Later on, the bottom notes will emerge and give you an indication of the perfume's depth and staying power. Inhale deeply (you can close your eyes if you want to – it's quite impressive), leaving at least thirty seconds or even a minute before trying the next. Let your nose rest a while, and then go back for another sniff test on all three. By this time you'll have probably been bombarded with facts about them, which you can sift through yourself.

Decisions, Decisions!

Don't ask the salesperson's opinion. She's not going to be wearing them, and anyway, her own preferences might not have much to do with yours. Remember also that she may have been told to push a certain line at the expense of others, so don't take too much notice of anything but essential information. It's you who has to make the choice, and you know your tastes better than she does.

Now that you've smelt the perfumes, ideally you should walk away from the whole environment. It's so easy to be seduced by the perfume counter and linger on, but don't: it will only cloud your decisions. The idea of walking away is to let the perfumes bloom to their fullest. If the salesperson is a good one she'll understand, or even suggest it. If you like, sleep on it. If you've been given strip samples, take them home and smell them now and then. Don't leave this too long, however, because they will fade pretty rapidly once exposed to air. You might end up not liking any of them, or one or two may be close to your target.

Before you take the plunge and choose which perfume you want, there a couple more things you have to consider. Firstly, money. A new perfume is a considerable outlay, and if you make a mistake there's no way of getting a refund once the bottle has been opened. At the top end of the market prices don't differ all that much from perfume to perfume. Perfumes on special are often excellent buys and are usually marked down because a new packaging or size is appearing. The old stock, unless it's really battered or the stopper is a bit dicey, should be perfectly okay.

The second choice you must make, and one which is tied to the issue of cost, is what strength you want. I firmly believe that the *extrait* or concentrated perfume is the best buy. Despite the initial financial outlay, not only is it stronger, it will last longer simply because you won't need to use so much of it. It is also much truer to what the perfume is *really* about. The lighter versions will come in various sizes, either in spray or splash form, and will be somewhat cheaper. They give you a faithful interpretation of the basic perfume, but of course don't have the same effect or endurance on the skin. The ideal is to have both concentrate and *eau de parfum* or *eau de toilette* if your budget can stretch to it. And do remember that, although perfume seems terribly expensive, when you break it down to how many applications for how many cents you get from one bottle, you may be pleasantly surprised. Of course it's not cheap, but then again, you don't want to smell cheap either!

Assuming you've got through this ordeal and made at least one successful choice, get to know your new love. By all means display it on your dressing table, but never under any circumstances leave it out of its protective box. The light will penetrate the glass and the perfume will discolour and gradually turn sour. If something happens to the box, secrete the carefully stoppered bottle upright in a very dark drawer or cupboard.

Now to the question of how to wear your perfume for maximum effect on others and maximum pleasure to yourself. It's a pity we can't spray perfumes on fabric, because it's there they will last longer. But, of course, they'll also stain your garment. Your pulse-points are the best carriers, since perfume will rise with body heat and surround you more quickly and lastingly. The V in your collarbone, between your breasts, the insides of your elbows, backs of your knees and the inside of your wrists are the best spots (don't, by the way, rub your wrists together thinking you'll achieve greater impact. All you'll do is crush the perfume's delicate stages of development). Behind the ears and on your temples and along the hairline are also good vantage points. A great idea is to dab or spray perfume onto little wads of cotton wool and secrete these in your bra, a pocket or in your purse, or even dab them along your arms and legs. Then there's the old trick of spraying the perfume in front of you and simply walking into it to give you an all-over envelopment.

Don't be afraid to apply your perfume confidently. As Coco Chanel once wisely said, 'A woman should wear her perfume where she wants to be kissed.' Simple as that.

THE
PERFUMES

An A to Z of the greats

This is where I take you on a tour of inspection of a whole lot of perfumes available for your choosing – the beauteous, the breathtaking, the brilliant, the bizarre, all of them extraordinarily diverse and with their own unique personalities. Amidst this august assemblage of perfumes, through the descriptions I have made of them, you may uncover some secrets about your favourite fragrances, or maybe you'll even discover some new perfume to suit you.

Not every perfume has been described here. Some have been made obsolete, never to be manufactured again. Others are so esoteric that I could not possibly have done them justice. Others again are so difficult to buy that I've felt it pointless to frustrate your efforts by including them. In the case of those perfumes I have not described but which you wish to track down, I suggest you do your own detective work with perfume outlets (you can usually order in a perfume from a department store or perfume boutique), the distributors or manufacturers. I have not indicated the various formulations, sizes and prices involved – these tend to change without warning, and the salesperson is your best help here.

My aim in this section has been to encapsulate each perfume – its type, its ingredients, its effect, its ambience, its pleasures and its magic. To me, perfume is more than an inanimate liquid in a bottle. It is a great constellation of earthly loveliness captured from the most beautiful smells on our planet in all their infinite variations.

Deciphering the ingredients with a reasonable amount of accuracy has sometimes been difficult when not too much information has been available. Therefore I've had to hazard a guess or two on occasion, so forgive me if I've sometimes made a mistake!

Let's now begin our scented journey, wandering down familiar avenues, turning a few surprising corners, being awestruck by some wonderful vistas, and hopefully not ending up in a *cul-de-sac*. I hope you will find it a fascinating stroll. Please do it in leisurely stages. Don't try to cover too much at once – you might overdose on opulence! But I do trust you'll come out at the end of it feeling and smelling as if you owned the world.

Bon voyage!

Alliage
by Estée Lauder

**PRONUNCIATION: alley-ARZJHE
ESS-tay LOR-da**

*a*lliage is French for 'alloy' or 'mixture', but I think it was the beautiful sound of the word, rather than its meaning, that must have recommended it to Lauder when the company launched its 'sport' perfume in 1972.

Like most green perfumes, you'll either like or loathe **Alliage**. It's a hugely uncompromising perfume, and fearless in its nose-thumbing, which extends even to its fellow greenies. For a start, with the exception of a very quick whiff of jasmine, it ignores flowers altogether and even goes easy on the woods. There's no sweetness in it, no attempt to soften the blow of strong green harmonies with their audacious quantities of nutmeg and citrus oils. Its basic note is galbanum, a strong green sap from the Middle East that is both sharp and pungent. To this is added a zesty crush of green leaves and citrus, before the middle note of nutmeg adds its characteristic haunting spiciness. This is pretty strong stuff, immediately steering the mix in a most adventurous and assertive direction, which turns out to be the forest floor, where oakmoss from the Balkans and vetyver from Java are taken on board to give a soft, almost musty, mossy pervasion.

Alliage isn't heavy but it *is* insistent. Its evergreen spirit is perfectly aligned to people possessing a sense of fun, of competitiveness, and with an uncomplicated attitude. All-American, you might say. It is hyperactive, tenacious and very compelling in its unorthodox way. In the Lauder line-up it's not madly popular but has a devoted clientele who prefer its dry honesty to the hotbeds of over-cultivated sophistication.

What to wear it with, where and when

Anything green (except a ballgown), in any shade. It's also great with white, yellow, mustard, curry, orange, sienna and grey, but no black, red, blue, purple, gold or silver. **Alliage** likes clothes it can relax in – unelaborate, with a minimum of decoration to concentrate on dashing simplicity. Cotton, linen, chambray, denim, georgette, organza and leather are its textures, and anything outdoors is its playground, although it can be worn indoors in casual company. It's essentially a young to young-forties perfume, wonderful in the heat of the day but a flop at night. Never wear it in winter – it smells perverse.

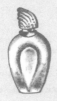

Amarige
by Givenchy

PRONUNCIATION: a m - a r - E E Z J H E
z j h i v - O N - s h e

Smelling **Amarige** for the first time is like walking through a dense, dripping jungle to be suddenly confronted by a flower so beautiful, so vivid, and with a scent so permeating, it stops you dead in your tracks. I don't know if there's such a word as 'amarige' in the French language, but I suspect it's been coined from *mariage*, French for marriage. And if this is the case, then **Amarige** is *some* wedding!

The composition itself is a departure from the conventional alliance of jasmine and rose, and the guests at the wedding are far from being bourgeois relatives. Although there is some jasmine present at the proceedings, it's very much in the back pews. The pervasive presence in the bouquet is unmistakably gardenia, but here transformed into a softer version of itself by being placed against exotic woods, most notably Brazilian rosewood with its deeply mellow smell. This is surrounded by lovely orange-smelling neroli, honeyed mimosa, sultry ylang ylang, and the elegance of violet. It's an exquisite bridal bouquet in which the gardenia shines through with a surprisingly subtle radiance.

'Sultry' is probably the word to describe this strong, elaborate and passionate perfume. 'Sumptuous' also comes to mind. Its unconventionality and its breeding place it well above the usual shriek and clamour of reckless 'moderns'. A woman will either fall immediately in love with it or avoid its uncompromising demands. It's a lusciously exotic perfume – mesmerising and sophisticated. It is Givenchy's most daring adventure.

What to wear it with, where and when

Take your colour inspiration from its brightly shining packaging – blood red, heliotrope, yellow, azure, emerald. These vibrantly outspoken colours are **Amarige**'s territory. It loves dazzle in fabrics, design and atmospherics. Parties are its natural hunting-ground, and it's something of a lethal weapon in the bedroom. You could successfully open a flower show in it, but don't wear it to the office unless you're the boss! The young to mature woman who is worldly-wise and sophisticated will gravitate towards it. Like **Amarige** itself, she will be elegantly individual, cultivated and quite calculating.

Anaïs Anaïs
by Cacharel

PRONUNCIATION: an-ASE an-ASE

cash-ar-EL

St Matthew tells us that Jesus, when considering the lilies of the field, proclaimed that even King Solomon in all his glory couldn't hold a candle to their beauty. And **Anaïs Anaïs**, with its intense concentration of lilies, is certainly a beauty.

Although too complex to be put into the single flower category, its bouquet is dominated by the rich, smooth and creamy scent of lilies, lilies and more lilies. Now too many lilies can be a touch overpowering, so Cacharel's perfumers have woven around them a garland of jasmine, white roses and irises, with hints of vetyver grass, a whiff of powerhouse patchouli and an acerbic spike of greenery to gild the lily, so to speak. In doing so, **Anaïs Anaïs** achieves a softness and subtlety that is utterly spellbinding, and will never bring on the vapours.

Apparently named after Anaitis, an ancient Persian love goddess, this hypnotic perfume is deceptively light, remaining softly persistent as it gradually and gracefully fades away. Incurable romantics will be captivated by its aura of nostalgic sighs and wistful longings.

Prettily packaged in white porcelain cylinders and featuring the Cacharel floral motif, it's a delight to give or receive and looks suitably shy on the dressing-table. **Anaïs Anaïs** is for the easily enamoured young sybarite, so even if you're more of a born-again virgin than the real thing, you can get away with it. But beware! If you're nearing that dreaded hill, or if you're already over it, give **Anaïs Anaïs** a wide berth. You might smell like mutton dressed up as lamb!

What to wear it with, where and when

White, silver, pink, pastels – definitely nothing strident or vivid, and in fabrics that are light, flimsy and diaphanous. Good with big cartwheel hats, little lace gloves, white stockings, strings of aquamarines and amethysts. Spring and summer are its perfect seasons. It's lovely floating on afternoon or evening air, and irresistible at twilight! Wear it to casual occasions with a romantic bent: tea parties, intimate dinners, Christenings and weddings – especially if you're the bride.

Armani
by Giorgio Armani

PRONUNCIATION: JAW-jee-o arrr-MAR-nee

*T*his perfume is perhaps not quite what you'd expect from the minimalist Italian designer who ruthlessly pares his clothes down to the essentials of a casual classicism that women adore. Armani's theory is that a perfume is an abstraction . . . a mystique. This certainly complements his stance on clothes but, amazingly, not in this his signature perfume.

Armani is flagrantly, unashamedly Italianate in its vivacious outspokenness. It is a perfume which comes straight to you rather than you having to make overtures to it, and it doesn't feel particularly obliged to take you on a labyrinthine journey to reveal its complexities either. It simply envelops you in the centre of its loveliness and commands you to revel in its lushness. There's no standing on ceremony, no gracious formality. It is an instant, spontaneous celebration of itself – like throwing a big impromptu party just for the hell of it!

To say that **Armani** is disarmingly sweet is something of an understatement. It is *very* sweet and quite tenacious, but not cloying. Its edges are soft, shadowy and seductive. This comes from its positive volley of glorious flowers. At first encounter there's a swooping onslaught of high-pitched greenery and soaring assaults of jasmine, rose, lily of the valley and hyacinth. These are backed with shots of coriander, basil and chypre with sandalwood and vetyver. All this is gathered together with musk to detonate an explosion, giving it its formidable staying power. **Armani** is composed of over eighty essences, but the overall effect is seamless, spectacular and disarming – a total intoxication.

People gravitate towards **Armani**. Wear it and you'll be bombarded with questions as to its intense identity. If you can, tell them nothing. Simply smile enchantingly and enigmatically and pretend you've quite forgotten its name.

What to wear it with, where and when

Armani is not strictly an 'occasion' perfume, but do be careful not to wear it to something too low-key; it will assert itself too much. It really is best at glittering parties where people will be disturbed by its loveliness. **Armani** happily attaches itself to any colour and it doesn't care about seasons either. It's at its most spectacular with quite extravagant or adventurous clothes that stand out in a crowd. As for moments in the boudoir, wear it carefully – just a subtle drop. It loves to be loved, but only if you're over twenty and under fifty.

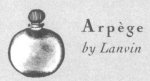

Arpège
by Lanvin

PRONUNCIATION:
ar-PAI-zjhe (as in 'beige')
lon-VAN

What a perfect name, chosen by Jeanne Lanvin's daughter to describe the almost indescribable quality of this grand classic. Translated as *Arpeggio*, a musical term for a rapid succession of upward notes, **Arpège** is an ecstatic, rapturous miracle.

Created by André Frayse for the House of Lanvin in 1927, when Madame Lanvin was at the peak of her career as a *couturière,* the perfume created quite a stir, being one of the cheeky new breed to use aldehydes as part of its complex composition. During the course of its life **Arpège** underwent a few slight tamperings, subtly but tellingly altering its smell. I am glad to report that at last this nonsense has been stopped and we are back to the amazingly original formula! Its newly restored classicism is impervious, and time has certainly not diminished its aura of elegant hauteur.

A gently outgoing perfume, it is a captivating *mélange* of opulent flowers seamlessly interwoven with woody, musky notes and a hint of sparkling green in its depths. It begins its chordal adventure with sweet Grasse jasmine and

Bulgarian rose, then builds up with contrapuntal themes of greener flower notes such as hyacinth and lily of the valley for a crisp freshness. Then comes the audacious introduction of heady, wild honeysuckle. An overlay of amber and musk with touches of vetyver and sandalwood culminate in a crescendo of intensely warm, autumnal radiance – very like Chopin at his most ardent and passionate!

Refinement is the word I associate with **Arpège** – a beautifully rounded composition with cultivated nuances and wild depths. In its gold-stoppered black orb bottle, it's been famous since its creation. But whatever you treasure it for, **Arpège** is a tirelessly romantic triumph, a masterpiece of balance, harmony, richness and, above all, opulent loveliness – a glorious, headlong rush of magical notes to be played over and over and over . . .

What to wear it with, where and when

Arpège is at its best with tailored or draped clothes – a smart town suit, a stunning little black dress, an arresting but unfussy evening bombshell. It cares not for seasons or ages, gliding with innate elegance and assurance through the years, giving away no secrets. **Arpège** adores refined reds, rich earth colours, lush cream and ivory, imperial purple, parma violet, copper, gold, and especially black. Being a Great Lady, it should be treated with a sense of refinement, so always look your best when you wear it.

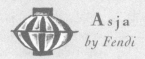

Asja
by Fendi

One look at the arresting gold-and-black-striped oval bottle and there'll be no prizes for guessing that this is an oriental! It seems that one of the formidable Fendi sisters, Carla, was wandering through Japan's Imperial Palace one fine day when she came upon a seventeenth-century porcelain bowl emblazoned with what looked exactly like the Fendi signature stripes. She was so entranced by its beauty, its compact shape and its sense of mystery that she set about creating what was eventually to be the lovely **Asja**.

It's a perfume likened to an escape into the unknown pleasures of the inscrutable Orient – enigmatic, sensual, disturbing, intimate. Just drawing the fire-red glass bottle from within the outer bowl is something of a thrill; this will clearly be a rivetingly different perfume. And **Asja** doesn't let you down. It's an opulent, splendid knockout, with haunting fruits, flowers and spices quite unlike the usual jasmine, rose and cinnamon journeys of its competitors.

Its magnetism begins with blackcurrant buds mixed with luscious fruits, sharp citrus accents, and what seems like an entire bazaar of fabulous flowers – Egyptian jasmine, dark Bulgarian roses, haunting ylang ylang and dazzling mimosa. Then the spice caravan arrives laden with cinnamon, nutmeg and cloves, each adding its dusky arabesque to those other oriental indispensables – sandalwood, musk, amber and vanilla.

The entire adventure is intoxicating. **Asja** seems to have found an enviable balance between volatile exotica and tranquil splendour, so subtle it never tips over into synthetic seductiveness or blatant vulgarity. It is as far from the clamour of the west as you can get, yet its eastern wiles are genuinely fascinating. One erstwhile journalist I read described it as 'a delicate floral oriental'. Delicate? Rubbish! Imperious is the word to describe **Asja**!

What to wear it with, where and when

Imagine you're an empress in ancient China swathed in red and saffron silk, or an Indian Maharani robed in gold and purple saris weighed down with precious jewellery, and you've got the **Asja** drift. Clothes should be simple but dramatic – more memorable than merely spectacular. Casual wear or anything 'cleverly' coordinated just isn't *de rigueur*. This makes it rather more of an occasion perfume than one you'd wear shopping. It's also more of an evening enchantment than a daytime one, so don't bother with it at lunch. Being a child of Fendi, it requires women of elegance and poise with a definite sense of theatre for its pervasive and persuasive purposes, so if you're a simple soul or under twenty, forget it!

Bal à Versailles
by Jean Desprez

PRONUNCIATION: bahl-ah-vair-SIGH
zjhon des-PRAY

*A*lthough it was created in 1962 – almost a youngster in classic perfume terms – this magnificent aristocrat is already hallowed as one of the greats. **Bal à Versailles** isn't a perfume to be trifled with. It was born to adorn the woman with an innate and unswerving love of luxury and good taste, a true individualist who realises the power of subtlety and, above all, radiates an elusive elegance.

Its composition is quite curious, considering its success and dedicated use by devotees. Although it might evoke images of the heady air at the Versailles Palace during the period of Louis XIV, the first whiff dashes any notions of it being frivolous and shallow. Even though it's blithely haughty, even unapproachable in many ways, it has a warmly enveloping aura that exudes self-confidence and a supremely refined gentility.

Basically, it's an opulent floral combination of jasmine from Italy and Egypt, with Turkish and Bulgarian roses and Moroccan orange flowers. But in the final result you'd be hard pressed to isolate any of these beauties, because over them comes a mysterious veil of the orient's most smouldering and sensuous offerings. Sandalwood dominates in combination with civet, golden amber, dashes of pervasive patchouli, musk and vetyver, sensual vanilla, resinous opoponax and interweavings of clove-scented carnation and heady acacia. What an avalanche of exotica!

Bal à Versailles is an intricate and unique creation, mysterious and incredibly haunting. It claims to contain over three hundred ingredients, so it shouldn't come as any great surprise to find it's more than a touch expensive. But it has such a powerful and tenacious effect that a bottle of the *extrait* or even the finely balanced *eau de toilette* will last you a long time. I think it's worth every cent!

What to wear it with, where and when

Swirls of silk, satin, brocade, lace or velvet, heavily embroidered or opulently printed, in darkly jewelled colours – garnet, tourmaline, amethyst and emerald – and definitely black, with lashings of old gold. To reveal the full splendours of **Bal à Versailles**, wear it early to late evening. It's not comfortable in broad daylight, but is permissible at a very intimate and smart luncheon engagement. Winter or summer, it never loses its dark dazzle and refined pleasures. This perfume is for the mature to the very mature only, and only for those with infinite taste and innate grace.

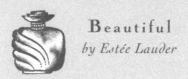

Beautiful
by Estée Lauder

*F*ortunately for **Beautiful** it is just that. For it to have been anything less would have been a disaster, but Estée Lauder is too clever by half. While non-American women may find the bulk of American perfumes a touch too strident, with **Beautiful**, Lauder almost (repeat, *almost*) errs on the side of comparative understatement. Despite its first rush of floral splendour, it is more softly spoken than most of its home-grown rivals. While its claim of 'smelling like a thousand flowers' might seem a bit extravagant, **Beautiful** is a splendidly floral artifice possessed of great lyrical charm.

It is composed of a very generous *mélange* of Bulgarian roses, French carnations, Moroccan and Egyptian jasmine, violets, orange blossom and delicate lily of the valley. Under this avalanche of sweetness is an earthy background of vetyver and thyme for a herbaceous and dusky quality, with the oriental scent of olibanum and the tenacious cling of musk. These notes tend to take away the voluptuous, heady edge from the rush of flowers while allowing them to exude their loveliness, as if they were filtered through spicy greenery. It's all very romantic, as intended.

Beautiful, like all pretty things, doesn't plumb the complex depths of subtlety like the great classic floral perfumes, but its feminine tenacity, although gentle and genteel, is vivacious, fresh and youthful. It's typically American in approach, all scrubbed-clean and wholesomely pert. As Mrs Lauder says, Beautiful is her tribute to vitality, youthful anticipation and hopeful beginnings. 'It's simply beautiful,' she says. But beauty being in the eye (and nose) of the beholder, Beautiful will either smell like a bed of roses to some, or an overdose of sweet sentimentality.

What to wear it with, where and when

'Think pink' and you're home and hosed with Beautiful. Cerise and cyclamen, hot pink and pretty pink, rose and fuchsia, powder pink and shocking pink – these shades, plus white and all the pastels, are ideal. Definitely no black! Beautiful is a knockout on brides and bridesmaids and is great at dances, parties and other exuberant social gatherings. Don't expose it to sporting occasions – it's more of a hothouse hybrid than an outdoors wildflower. It's also for the young only – nobody pushing thirty should dare to get away with it. Of course it blooms at its prettiest in spring.

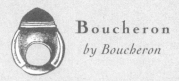

Boucheron
by Boucheron

*T*he birth of **Boucheron** reads like the highest of high dramas. Alain Boucheron, head of the jewellery empire of the same name, was about to launch his super-expensive brainchild into the top end of the perfume market when he had a last sniff of the stuff to make sure everything was bang-on. He took a long whiff and, *quelle horreur!*, instinctively knew that all was not right: the top note was too aggressive. So, at the last minute, he had the formula changed to make it smoother and more elegant. **Boucheron** was subsequently launched to great acclaim.

God knows what the original top note was because the new ones – tangerine, orange and apricot – are pretty powerful anyway. They hold their forthright stance for quite a while before allowing any of the other ingredients to make an entrance. Eventually, through the pure golden blaze, the scent of jasmine emerges, backed by the richness of ylang ylang. Then subtle notes of orange blossom, tuberose and narcissus filter harmonically through to make the heart of the perfume elegantly feminine without being over-romantic or sentimental. Tenderness and persuasion are not **Boucheron**'s intentions. It is too assertive and well mannered to be considered intimate, but it's the base notes of amber and particularly tonka bean that give it its final substance and depth.

This is the sort of self-assured perfume you'd expect from the undisputed ruler of jewellery design. Its ritz is splendid but refined, its clout quite emphatic. Contained in a sapphire and gold ring bottle, it looks like a precious and beautiful jewel. One must admit that it amply fills Monsieur Boucheron's strategy of achieving 'permanent synergy' between jewellery and perfume. But I can't help wondering what the original top note was, and what **Boucheron** *might* have been – aggression and all!

What to wear it with, where and when

La crème de la crème is the natural stamping ground of this rather haughty and aloof perfume. The very best fabrics, beautifully handled and cut, are necessary for its ambience. Moving as it does in a world of jewels, the jewel colours are completely *simpatico* with its quiet grandeur – particularly the warmer blazes of tourmaline, topaz, amber and, of course, gold. However, since it is almost its own jewel, don't weigh yourself down with glamour and glitter – too much of anything is anathema to its refined stance. Leave it at home through the day; it really is an occasion perfume and holds its own quite civilly among the 'screamers' which shrink at its grand credentials. Don't let the kids near it, though – it will eat them alive! And you can wear it all year round; it won't wilt, but it will fight with the gardenias.

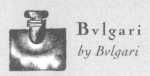

Bvlgari
by Bvlgari

*I*n the wake of Van Cleef & Arpels, Boucheron, Cartier and Tiffany, it was inevitable that this great Italian jewellery house would enter the perfume field with its own eponymous dazzler. It had a few great acts to follow, but when it comes to opulent splendour, the House of Bvlgari is no slouch.

Bvlgari is a perfume that wins by sheer beauty – the kind of beauty that simply invades you with its exquisite loveliness and refinement. It arrives in a striking bottle that is half-transparent, half-frosted, and topped by an austere gold cap. It exudes not just good, but *impeccably* good, taste. The perfume approaches you with a sumptuous bouquet of flowers arranged with great ingenuity. You will detect jasmine and orange blossom, then hints of ylang ylang and mimosa. Roses are embedded as well, but not just any rose – **Bvlgari** uses the wonderful Prelude rose for the very first time in perfume, giving the bouquet a sweet subtlety with a joyous high note. But the surprises aren't over yet!

There's the rich rainforest smell of Brazilian rosewood, vetyver, Florentine iris and musk to add depth. Out of all this sings the very clear note of violet.

Then, when you think the gentle seduction is complete, the *coup d'eclat* is delivered with rare sleight of hand: the imaginative infusion of Sambac jasmine-scented green tea, of all things! Don't expect to suddenly get a whiff of an exotic teabag or even a few tannic leaves. **Bvlgari** is too tasteful for such cheap tricks. Instead, you get the impression of a slightly green and oriental waft to give a final edge to the perfume. It doesn't stand out and assault you, but whispers and haunts, so that finally **Bvlgari** leaves you with a sense of mystery and serenity – and that little touch of extravagance it is sometimes impossible to resist.

What to wear it with, where and when

Bvlgari loves clothes and colours that are feminine without being fussy. Muted or shaded rose colours, hazy purples, cloudy yellows, cream and magnolia, dark emerald green and indigo are its natural complements, in fabulous fabrics like silk and satin, taffeta and brocade, chiffon and georgette, even lace. Occasions can be grand or low-key, though not *too* humble. I wouldn't advise wearing **Bvlgari** outdoors either – fresh air would offend its pedigree! Age is neither here nor there, nor season. It is not a snobby or haughty perfume, and therefore behaves with impeccable manners at all times.

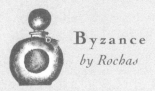

Byzance
by Rochas

*E*ast meets west in a perfect accord of flowers, fruits, woods and spices in this alluring and ultra-feminine perfume. As its name suggests, **Byzance** is an evocation of Byzantium, the fabled city built by the Greeks. Like the city, it is neither occidental nor oriental but a true Middle Eastern melding, a *mélange* of fascinating facets.

While its name is redolent of a fabulous world of inspired art and architecture, **Byzance** is not as serious and heavy a smell as you might expect. In fact, it's quite light and luminous, with none of the raunchy aspects of the Turkish bazaar. Its beauty begins with its glorious bottle – a spectacular deep electric-blue orb emblazoned with a bold gold label and stoppered with a smooth, blue glass dome, all tied with dark cyclamen braids. Its composition is an intricate mosaic of both eastern and western flowers – rose, jasmine, lily of the valley and white stock (which accounts for its clove-like spiciness). For fruit it features Mediterranean mandarin, plus musk and vanilla and the soft glow of sandalwood to round out its tantalising message. But the modern cleverness of the Occident has the last say with a hushed overlay of soft chemical aldehydes, giving **Byzance** its glowing sheen and patina of glamour.

It's a beautifully balanced fantasia of sweetness and sparkle, sensuousness and opulence, played with lightly suggestive nuances rather than a blaze of trumpets from the minaret. Women who prefer to entice and fascinate will understand its arabesque persuasions.

What to wear it with, where and when

The beautiful jewel colours of the bottle itself are the clues to successfully wearing **Byzance**. Don't wear anything remotely busy or tizzy with it, and nothing obviously *femme fatale* either. It loves velvet, silk, taffeta, fur, organza, lamé and superfine wool, in clothes of flowing cut and line – things that look sensuous but languid. It loves swish parties, banquets and balls, as well as super-expensive restaurants and anywhere with lots of light and laughter. The young can wear it quite charmingly, but it's the mature and very mature who understand its subtle wiles instinctively.

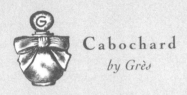

Cabochard
by Grès

*I*n case you didn't know, *cabochard* literally means 'pig-headed, wilful, obstinate', but the French, being elastic about these matters, usually take it to mean something less abrasive: 'charmingly persistent'.

This mysterious perfume was created in 1958 after Madame Grès experienced the myriad magics of India. As a result, **Cabochard** has a distinct aura of that subcontinent, making it more specific than a generic oriental. Although the basis of it is a heady blend of exotic flowers, spices, woods and animal notes, the most striking presence to my nose is Indian patchouli. In the classicist hands of Madame Grès this much-misused ingredient is indeed 'charmingly persistent', giving point and accent to the other components which overlay it. These are many and varied – roses and jasmine for richness, oakmoss for soft greenness, carnation for spicy sweetness, hyacinth for delicacy, citrus oils for sharpness, a forest of woods, including sandalwood, rosewood and vetyver grass for warmth, a hint of Russian leather to give a burnished opulence, and some very evident animal notes from musk, civet and ambergris.

Thus **Cabochard** has an enigmatic but highly distinctive character. It never succumbs to the wild or uncivilised, much less lustier aspects of oriental persuasions. Indian by inspiration it may be, but Parisian it most certainly is in demeanour. Yet its secret weapon, under all its Parisian poise, is its unexpected chicanery. It's quite a little devil, so don't underestimate its powers.

Cabochard is not as ubiquitous as it once was, but in its chunky, cheeky little bottle with a frosted glass stopper and a grey velvet bow adorning its neck, it's still a symbol of refined and dignified sophistication – with that Indian exoticism lurking and smouldering just below the surface.

What to wear it with, where and when

If you've ever drooled over photographs of the beautifully sculpted, draped and pleated classic Greek columns of a Grès dress, you'll know instinctively what to wear with this perfume and how to wear it. **Cabochard** needs the grace and elegance of lovely, flowing fabrics such as silk jersey, chiffon, silk, velvet and crêpe. It's also a knockout with smart, tailored clothes – city suits, snappy cocktail dresses (including the little black number). Its colours are gregarious – from grey, mushroom, beige, cream and white through to mysterious greens, blues, muted yellow, powdery pink, deep rose, heliotrope and lots of black. Seasons aren't important to its mysterious blooming, but it's best in the late afternoon or evening. For the mature and very mature, but only if they are elegance personified.

Cabotine
by Grès

A fair word of warning: if you're over the age of twenty-five, forget **Cabotine**. As perfumes go, they don't come any younger or more spirited than this beguiling gamine.

It's high time the young and lively were catered for with a perfume that seems exclusively made for them. There's not much around that can be called totally young in attitude; perhaps **Miss Dior**, **Diorissimo**, **Anaïs Anaïs**, **Loulou**, **L'Air du Temps**, **Jicky**, **Je Reviens**, **Moschino** and **Pleasures** just about fill the slim bill, but they can be equally captivating on older women as well. **Cabotine** isn't.

As the advertisement for it says, it's *'un parfum presque innocent'*, meaning almost innocent. It's a bit of a flirt – a naughty, unpredictable little minx who nevertheless is disarmingly charming. Its fragrance is not reticent or bashful; rather it's strong, sweet and extremely tenacious. Its floral basis is an imaginative accord of white ginger lily and tuberose, the tropical lushness of one balancing the heady romanticism of the other. Add to this white orange flowers, the zestiness of mandarin and lime, the soft sigh of sandalwood clinging together with sensuous musk, and that gives you an idea of the game **Cabotine** plays – very worldly indeed, yet professing wide-eyed innocence.

If Madame Grès, that unrivalled genius of swathed, draped *couture,* was still with us to enjoy the charm of **Cabotine**, she'd have been happy that the Acadamia del Profumo honoured it with the International Award for the Best Female Fragrance in 1992, a prize it richly deserves, especially for its squat little bottle sporting a knockout bow tie of emerald glass.

What to wear it with, where and when

From jeans and T-shirts through to frivolous little *décolleté* numbers, **Cabotine** shines, especially with light, bright colours – greens, blues, yellows, pinks and especially white. It's a perfume that loves craziness and invention, nothing conventional. It doesn't give a hoot whether it's day or night, and is so friendly and ingratiating it can go anywhere with confidence. It's an outrageous but irresistible flirt, especially in spring and summer.

Calandre
by Paco Rabanne

PRONUNCIATION: karl-ARND-ruh
PAH-ko rah-BAHN

*T*his one always reminds me of Joan Crawford in *Mildred Pierce*, racing around slapping people's faces, hard as nails, but underneath a softer heart beating passionately – misunderstood, mistreated, long-suffering but noble.

Calandre is steely on the outside but intensely romantic at heart. It's a perfume that's been ignored of late simply because it's been around for so long. Like Rabanne's lethal-looking *couture* of the late sixties, it caused quite a sensation at its launch. Uncompromising, daring and avant-garde, the fashion establishment shuddered and hoped the whole Rabanne thing would go away. But it didn't, and his perfume is still with us.

Calandre was the first floral aldehyde perfume to also feature a sharp green note of equal potency and still manage to maintain a distinctive clarity. It combines roses and jasmine, with the emphasis heavily on roses, then adds pungent modern aldehydes, the citrus sharpness of hesperides and a green trill that slashes through the floral sweetness like a razor-sharp scythe. I've even heard that the formula contains iron filings – a probability, given Rabanne's sense of adventure. (It could well explain the magnetic appeal of **Calandre**!)

Needless to say, this is a very assertive perfume, though not at all rough or aggressive. Its inherent dramatics are high-powered and emphatic, and it has an almost stark austerity. Despite this the discerning nose will discover that its real heart, the one that pounds with passion, is a bed of roses – intense, powerful and ultimately comforting.

What to wear it with, where and when

Calandre is one of those gifted perfumes that sails blithely and confidently through every season and temperature. It's an extemely versatile *accoutrement*, able to rise to grand occasions as well as fit comfortably into more intimate surroundings. It doesn't appeal to the very mature, working best on young sophisticates with a rather wild bent. Definitely a party girl, it shines in sensational short blacks, glittery silvers and platinums, coppers, golds, sheeny greys and greens. It's also dynamite with cobalt and shocking pink. Long, leggy girls just love it to death!

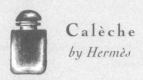

Calèche
by Hermès

*I*t's a soft and misty dawn in the Bois de Boulogne. The sharp clip-clop of horses' hooves echo in the still air as the *calèche*, driven by a liveried servant, travels homewards. The occupant of the carriage is a beautiful, veiled woman. An elegantly gloved hand lifts the veil to wipe away an errant tear of *joie* or *tristesse* – or both. She leans back against the silk upholstery and smiles mysteriously, wisely, wickedly . . .

Today's woman doesn't travel in a *calèche*; instead, she wears it! Although this hugely successful and greatly loved classic wears the lovely mantle of nostalgia for a bygone era, it's far from old hat or old-fashioned. Created in 1961, **Calèche** was the first perfume to come from the great leather-making House of Hermès. It is rich, refined and polished, with a burnished luxuriousness. It is also very assertive – a headlong rush of greens, flowers, spices and woods, all galloping furiously neck-and-neck.

It's difficult to pull this perfumed jigsaw apart, but the initial onslaught definitely comes from an acerbic jab of chypre sharpness tempered with oakmoss and bracing vetyver.

With this outdoor sting established, a procession of flowers is ushered in with a heady blaze of jasmine, gardenia, rose, iris and lily of the valley. After this thoroughbred entourage comes the zing of citrus oils and the airiness of orange blossom with an added dazzle of ylang ylang. Finally, a good dash of spice and a delicate veil of woods of pine, cedar and sandalwood bring an earthy touch to this brilliant, finely tuned masterpiece.

Calèche loves nothing more than the excitement of the moment – the sudden explosion of fireworks, the lure and impetuousness of a *liaison dangereuse*. It's provocative enough to tempt you to plunge into forbidden waters, so you too can sneak home triumphantly on a misty morning, just beating the dawn and harsh reality to the door!

What to wear it with, where and when

Calèche adores luxury but not silly extravagance or vulgarity. Fur, leather, suede, silk, velvet and lace are its night-time fabrics, and for daywear it is perfect with cashmere, alpaca, wool, jersey, linen and georgette. Clothes can be quite formal or casually chic as long as they're beautifully tailored or draped. Colours should be rich and earthy – subdued red, mustard, curry, cream and gold. **Calèche** is fine in all seasons and weathers, from daylight to dark, and gives off warm vibrations in the boudoir.

The
Caron Classics
by Caron

*T*he younger generation of perfume users may never have heard of this highly respected and visionary perfume house. Founded in the early years of the century by perfumer Ernest Daltroff, Caron has become synonymous with a legion of high-class creations.

Daltroff opened his perfume boutique in fashionable rue de la Paix in Paris, from where he launched in 1911 a dynamic perfume called **Narcisse Noir**. It caused a sensation in France, and Daltroff, instinctively anticipating its acceptance in America, quickly exported it there. With one single perfume his international reputation was forged.

His perfumes were given arresting names and bottled in magnificently unique containers. Fortunately, some of them have survived to give their individual brilliance to a world of perfumes that too often seem to copy each other.

Here I have listed some of the Caron classics that, with a bit of sleuthing, you may be able to track down. I must warn you, though, that they are mostly a formidable lot – they are 'love it or hate it' fragrances, and not one of them is for the faint-hearted or the timid.

Bellodgia

PRONUNCIATION: bell-ODGE-ee-ah

If you dote on the spicy, clove-like sweetness of carnations, you'll think you're in seventh heaven wearing **Bellodgia**. It's a marvellously romantic, richly exotic perfume. Although dominated by carnations, it is really a blend, with jasmine, spices and woods giving the carnations their lingeringly sweet charm. Strictly for spring and summer and best on the mature to the very mature, it's a perfume to lose your heart to.

Fleur de Rocaille

PRONUNCIATION: fler duh rok-EYE

This perfume was launched with great pride in 1933 and immediately declared the first great floral bouquet. A complex *mélange* of lilac, lily of the valley, jasmine, iris, violet and rose against a sunny backdrop of sandalwood, musk and civet, the great thing about it was its extraordinary delicacy, persistence and vivacity. Then, without warning, it disappeared; not only a mystery, but a loss. Only recently has it shyly reappeared. Having not been familiar with the original, I can't say whether or not it has been altered, but as it stands now it is still a very lovely, sweet composition. **Fleur de Rocaille** is an absolute must for the young – the over twenty-fives will just have to wish they could still get way with its endearing young charms!

Infini

PRONUNCIATION: an-fee-NEE

This is one of the newer Caron breed, having been created in 1970. It's a most uncommon perfume — a heady and potent mix of rose, jasmine, lily of the valley, tuberose and jonquil pitted one against the other in concentrations so intense it takes the presence of sandalwood and other exotic woods, plus a *bouquet garni* of herbs and spices, to stop the lot from becoming a rampage! Definitely only for the sophisticated woman, it's to be sternly avoided by the young. **Infini** might give them ideas well above their capacities!

Muguet du Bonheur

PRONUNCIATION: MEW-gay doo bon-ERR

Muguet is French for the beloved lily of the valley, that tender, tiny bell-flower so prized when it pops up every spring. Many, many perfumes would lose their cheeky but sweet piquancy without it. **Muguet du Bonheur**, however, was probably the original perfume to use it as the dominating fragrance. It is a radiantly evocative perfume that presents a glade of greenery through which the lily of the valley emerges with an almost heart-rending clarity and sweetness. Its cool, foresty call is sheer bliss in spring, which is why **Muguet du Bonheur** should not be worn by anyone past the springtime of their youth. However, it's so lovely you may think you've recovered yours.

Narcisse Noir

Narcisse Noir was the miracle that made Caron. When you smell this rebel, you can imagine what a sensation it must have caused in its day. A potent and explosive concentration of narcissus, bergamot and sandalwood with a flamboyant dash of spice thrown in, it is sensual, challenging and downright sexy. Wear it only in cool weather and only if you're over twenty-five. Even then you have to be the smouldering type to carry it off with panache!

Nocturnes

Nocturnes is exactly what its name implies – a romantic night perfume full of persuasion and promise. Launched in 1981, it is typical of the Caron penchant for creating smooth, rich floral bouquets underlined with tantalising spices. In its dramatic but sensuous black bottle, **Nocturnes** is a seductive charmer – a mesmerising *mélange* of rose, tuberose, jasmine and ylang ylang with the quiet tenacity of woods and the zing of spices peppering its lushness. Of all the Caron perfumes, it is the most overtly and proudly feminine, sending out its suggestive intimations as an invitation to something truly sensual. Don't worry about seasons, but make sure you wear it only when the sun has firmly set. And be subtle, please!

Nuit de Noël

PRONUNCIATION: nwee duh no-ELL

A perfume to celebrate Christmas night, but only if you're in the northern hemisphere. In other words, if you live in the antipodes, keep it for autumn and winter: it practically faints in summer heat! **Nuit de Noël** is composed of sultry, exotic woods with rich jasmine and roses and a bazaar-full of spices to give it its warm, smouldering, almost fruity sumptuousness. It's brave, arresting, challenging and ravishing, and it takes a highly individual woman to do justice to its rich but uncompromising ambience. Testament to its classicism is the fact that it's been with us since 1922 and has, as far as I know, never been totally unavailable. In its way, it's comparable to that other rich, worldly-wise beauty, Guerlain's **L'Heure Bleue**, but is even more unconventional! So, you've been warned.

Parfum Sacré

PRONUNCIATION: par-FUOM sark-RAY

Always a faithful guardian of the bastions of civilised elegance, Caron has done it again in creating the imposing **Parfum Sacré**. Sadly, this perfume hasn't met with a great deal of popular success since its recent launch, probably due to the fact that it's considered too opulent for today's sober lifestyles. But that doesn't mean it hasn't found a special niche in the perfume world.

Parfum Sacré is Caron's subtle homage to the enduring beauty of the rose. It's not an outright rose type, but one which shrouds the flower in order to reveal its depths and mysteries ever so gradually. It starts with pepper and a dash of coriander, then plunges you straight into the depths of myrrh and musk – a formidable alliance indeed! Myrrh itself has long been considered sacred, with its incense-and-licorice intensity and strong religious associations, and the permeating powers of musk are a fine foil for it. Then comes the triumphant infusion of *rose absolu* lavished with hints of jasmine, orange blossom and vanilla. The list of ingredients is now complete, and it all adds up to a deep, disturbing and penetrating perfume which, even at its most open, never fully reveals its haunting rose base. **Parfum Sacré** shuns the limelight to cast its spell over the privileged few destined to discover it. I hope you're one of the fortunate.

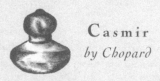

Casmir
by Chopard

The lotus blossom is a symbol of the fabled state of Kashmir, and that's almost how you pronounce this perfume's name, only with a soft whisper blurring the edges of the word. The lotus-shaped bottle, with its gold cap resembling the dome of the Taj Mahal, sends out the Indian message straight away.

Casmir is one of those oriental perfumes that, apart from a plethora of fabulous flowers, also delves deeply into the delectable use of luscious fruits. And it does so with a vengeance! It's romantic, sensuous, persuasive and erotic. At first whiff you are plunged into a complex cauldron of smouldering and succulent mango mixed with peach, coconut, hesperides and bergamot liberally laced with sensuous vanilla. The flowers then breathe romance into the proceedings – jasmine, lily of the valley and pungent geranium. Then there's an underscoring of amber, musk, more vanilla and castoreum, a warm, animalic scent with a long-lasting earthy note.

It's a very intricate fragrance, with no single note sounding a fanfare but instead presenting a strong impression of

Indian bazaars in their extraordinary accumulation of fascinating fragrances. **Casmir** is unabashedly oriental, but devotees of sensual exotica will want to be awash in its 'forbidden' fruits and flowers.

Be warned – **Casmir** is a highly individualistic and enigmatic perfume, nothing like the sweet and seductive delights of oriental charmers such as **Shalimar** or **Opium**. It smoulders darkly and mysteriously.

What to wear it with, where and when

You don't have to religiously wrap yourself in a gorgeous gold-spun sari, but anything resembling such oriental opulence is a good start. **Casmir** certainly favours rich silks, satins, all sheers and brocades, as well as leather and suede. Its best colours are earthy red-browns, copper, darkly intense reds, burnt orange, midnight blue, forest green, silvery grey, gold and black. It's not a daytime perfume – far too sonorous and sombre – but blooms at sundown or after it. It's a perfume I think that gives of its best in autumn or winter. And it's strictly for the twenty-fives and over, and then only if you have a touch of sensuality and earthiness. Definitely not for blue-eyed blondes!

Chamade
by Guerlain

PRONUNCIATION: shah-MARD
gair-LARN

What sort of perfume would you expect to find capturing the essence of this beautiful French word which, with typical Gallic ambivalence, can mean either 'the rapid beating of the heart' or 'the drumroll that signifies the moment of final surrender'? One of hot, unbridled passion? One that is all frenzy and fireworks? One that's an explosion of strong-scented flowers and spices?

Well, you get none of that from Guerlain's super-sensitive, rapturous, warm-hearted sensation. Emerging in 1969, **Chamade** had an extremely long gestation period. In trying to capture the 'utterly compelling moment of *chamade*', Jean-Paul Guerlain had 1300 cracks at it over seven years before he discovered exactly what he wanted. What eventuated was a perfume so gloriously different it all but redefined the meaning of the French word for the 'total surrender of the heart'.

If ever there was a perfume that creates its own beautifully serene orbit of persuasion it is **Chamade**. It insinuates rather than declaims, charms rather than flirts, floats rather than flashes. It is totally enigmatic yet totally approachable. Based on a mixture of natural oils and essences and enticing new aldehydes, **Chamade** emerges with enviable artistry. The synthetic input is used only to brighten and heighten the natural base which is a coming-together of Spanish lilac, hyacinth and tuberose. This intense trio is calmed with murmurs of jasmine, lily of the valley, vanilla and amber with a pungent whiff of cedar and some glowingly ripe fruits (mainly blackcurrant buds and plum), all magically held in a suspension of tropical oils.

Chamade is uniquely aloof but it knows how to persuade with a cultivated allure, an enveloping warmth and privacy, and just a touch of flirtatious but mature mischief.

What to wear it with, where and when

Chamade's softness can seduce you into thinking of mistily romantic clothes all wafting poetically about in the twilight when in actual fact it is the secret weapon of the prowling tigress! It loves richness, luxury, grandness and body heat. It dislikes being played down and demands to be worn with beautiful, softly cut clothes. Keep it lush but unfailingly ladylike in vibrant but not garish colours, not to forget white and black. Don't wear it everywhere but only unleash it when you feel very much in command and ready to purr! And you must be over twenty-five.

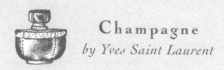

Champagne
by Yves Saint Laurent

PRONUNCIATION: shom-PINE-yeh
eve sarn-lor-ON

The French can be very perverse when something upsets them. The launch of Yves Saint Laurent's **Champagne** brought on a brouhaha of almost revolutionary proportions from the vignerons of Champagne itself. After all, they'd successfully battled American and Australian wine makers who had had the gall to call their sparkling whites by the exclusive name, so Saint Laurent's perfume was a sitting duck. The French courts ruled that it could no longer carry the exalted name.

So far Australia has been allowed to keep the label **Champagne**, even if the French haven't, but the question which must be asked is this: does the perfume live up to its august name?

From my point of view, I think **Champagne** has not only caught the glamour of the wine but also its ambience – not the smell or taste, of course, but the effect of it. Based on that luscious fruit, the nectarine, and composed of earthy ingredients such as *mousse de chine* (oakmoss), vetyver, patchouli, aniseed, mint and lychee with a typically Gallic dash of romantic country rose thrown in for good measure, **Champagne** is really a pastoral perfume. It isn't overpoweringly zingy or zesty; it doesn't tickle the nose and make you sneeze in giddy ecstasy. Rather, it's surprisingly refined and sophisticated in a low-key way.

In **Champagne** a new technique is used for extracting the essence of the fruits just before picking time to achieve a rather virginal radiance, a lushness and freshness that sings high and sweet. The clever alliance with rose and the chypre ingredients works fabulously with the nectarine deliciousness, and the hints of mint and aniseed are indeed inspired. It's not a fruit salad, however – more like a trembling fruit mousse.

If you're not naturally vivacious, no amount of **Champagne** will transform you into a glamorous hedonist. But for bubbling, burbling, ebullient and spirited souls, this is just the thing to keep your spark effervescing.

What to wear it with, where and when

Over-extravagance doesn't suit **Champagne** at all; it's too free-spirited and light for that. Wear it with well-cut casuals to chic luncheons, galleries, cocktail parties, non-first nights and informal dinners. **Champagne** likes chiffon, georgette, organza, cotton, crêpe, silk, suede, taffeta, lace and the odd sequin. For colours, it's a natural with orange, yellow, red, brown, cream, bright green and soft grey. I'd avoid all the blues, purple and dreamy pastels. It's fine in all seasons and covers a wide age spectrum as long as you join in the fun and get happily tipsy on its infectious effects.

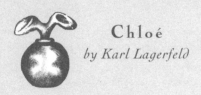

Chloé
by Karl Lagerfeld

PRONUNCIATION: KLO-ee
karl LARG-a-feld

When he took over the reins of Chanel in the seventies, Lagerfeld naturally caused quite an upheaval. To his credit he still does. The path to success, however, was rocky.

In 1975 when he launched the first perfume under his name, poor **Chloé** had more than her fair share of critics. The perfume was dismissed as being too heavy, too cloying, too sweet and too old-fashioned. Even the design of the bottle, with its soft curves and lily-shaped stopper, was criticised. Soon, however, its utter originality and unequivocal ambience began to reveal itself.

Lagerfeld's formulation is aimed directly at the heart. **Chloé** is a perfume of love – intimate, uninhibited, and passionate. If it is 'heavy', it's simply because it is absolutely committed to the exploitation of one dominant flower – the pervasively lovely tuberose. Tuberose is an unmistakable scent. It clings, it envelops, it persists and permeates, but it does all this with a rare beauty. Its scent is rich and creamy, almost euphoric, and when handled by a perfumer of great skill can be the ideal catalyst, the point of departure.

After the initial shock of the tuberose's volatility, other flowers begin to slowly surface in its wake – spring roses, night-scented jasmine, wild honeysuckle, and the haunting aureole of orange blossom. This exquisite blend is then softened and deepened against a wooded backdrop of oakmoss with a touch of patchouli, musk and amber. The total effect is nothing short of hypnotic.

Chloé is never claustrophobic but exhilarating and vivacious. To my mind it is a Botticelli-curved woman, soft and pliant, graceful and bending. It is all surrender.

What to wear it with, where and when

Pastels like dusky pink, powder blue, soft grey, muted green or anything flecked sparingly with gold are especially lovely with **Chloé**. So are white and cream and all the lilac shades. Clothes and fabrics should be filmy and draped or clean-cut and simple. **Chloé** is at its romantic best in late spring and summer, especially on afternoons under trails of weeping willows. But be sparing with it – too much of it will either bring on the vapours or frighten Prince Charming away!

Cinnabar
by Estée Lauder

**PRONUNCIATION: SINNA-bar
ESS-tay LOR-da**

*I*t was inevitable that Lauder would hitch itself to the oriental perfume caravan when it began its comeback journey in the mid to late seventies, and **Cinnabar** was its sophisticated passenger.

Like all of the Lauder perfumes, **Cinnabar** is smooth and svelte, despite its oriental heritage. In fact, it's a beautifully achieved interpretation of what many women imagine oriental perfumes to be. (The actual ones encountered in the Orient are far less ladylike, by and large!)

Cinnabar is not like deliberately losing yourself in the dangerous medina and hoping some romantic brigand will abduct you to his hideaway oasis. It is more like taking a guided tour of the bazaar in the company of venerated tribal elders. You can look your best, keep your cool, not be ripped off or carried off, and return to the sanctuary of your luxury hotel in one piece.

In composition it's a civilised harmony of warm fruits and romantic flowers, using exotic eastern potions to link the two. The four principal components are clove bud and citrus oils, strong jasmine absolute, and the mysterious-sounding olibanum, which is another name for frankincense. Add to these some soft floral aldehydes and the glow of amber and you have the recipe for a well-bred, sleek and fairly safe adventure.

Cinnabar is not in the least bland but always well mannered and fascinating. It's rather like donning a beautiful burnous of amber-coloured silk embroidered with delicate gold arabesques, letting your hair down in an elegant cascade, adorning yourself with silver and copper jewellery, and letting go – in the nicest possible way. You may not whip up a sandstorm, but you'll certainly be on a civilised sheik's most-desired list!

What to wear it with, where and when

Since 'cinnabar' means vermilion, use that colour as your guide to dressing. Vibrant reds, oranges, copper, amber, yellow, black, white, gold and even hot pink won't feel out of place. Cool blues and greens are also very nice with it, and so are neutrals, but leave the pretty pastels at home. **Cinnabar** suits loose, orientally inspired clothes in soft and sumptuous fabrics, but it also takes to high-class tailoring with touches of exotica. Plenty of chunky jewellery is almost mandatory. Brunettes and redheads are naturals for its calculated sense of adventure, and it should be worn at big occasions or very intimate ones, especially in the cooler seasons. It's for the mature and worldly-wise, and although not totally X-rated, you may need to approach it with more than a touch of caution.

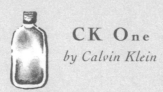

CK One
by Calvin Klein

I think **CK One** was created to summarise the nineties. Aligning itself with the politically and socially correct safeties of the times, it makes no great statement, thus offending no one. It does not prohibit either sex but is careful to point out it is no silly, old-fashioned 'unisex' perfume. It knows no boundaries but doesn't tear down any real walls, and it doesn't discriminate when it comes to a person's age. It is all things to all people – as long as they're honest, open and natural.

CK One is really a quite simple affair – pleasant, clean, clear, uncomplicated and exuberant. You can splash it all over you or dab it here and there whenever you will. It's not in the least tenacious, so it doesn't come on strong. The publicist of **CK One** claims it does what no other fragrance has done before – it 'makes you free'.

Certainly it's bright and light enough to go with your sense of newly acquired liberation. Right from the top it sparkles with bergamot and some sweet-spiced cardamom, plus fresh pineapple and papaya to keep it in the current trend of fruity fragrances. Its centre has an intriguing core of hedione high cis, a special formulation derived from jasmine. It uses this in very high concentration, allowing the attendant notes of violet, rose and nutmeg to be more intensified without overstepping the mark and upstaging their companions. Also evident is a fascinating accord of green tea — another very 'in' variant used in these types of lighter-than-light fragrances. The finish is rounded off with two varieties of musk and some sensuous amber.

CK One is only an *eau de toilette*, but it comes in a body massage and soothing lotion as well for that all-over feel-good message. To say that it is a fragrance that's neither here nor there would be unfair. It certainly makes its mark with those people, male or female, who don't want to smell too obvious but feel unfinished without a light and hip fragrance.

What to wear it with, where and when

Treated in much the same way as the indestructable **No. 4711**, or any other straight *cologne*, you can't go too far wrong. **CK One** will fit in anywhere, any time, when worn by practically anyone. It's not something you'd make a great fuss over as far as colours, clothes or special occasions go. It's not meant for grandeur, and I doubt if you'd be successful with it as part of a grand strategy of seduction either. Just use it where you will, winter or summer, day or night, whether you're eighteen or eighty, male or female. It fits in with any lifestyle. Who could ask for anything more?

Coco
by Chanel

PRONUNCIATION: shar-NEL

I don't know if Madame Chanel would have quite approved of having her *sobriquet* attached to this perfume, which appeared many, many years after her death. She always guarded her private image ferociously and looked down on all efforts to emulate her personal style. But somehow I think she would have been quite flattered by **Coco**.

This outspoken, freewheeling and ravishing perfume is loved by a lot of women. After its huge launch in 1985 it became obvious that **Coco**'s creator, the great perfumer Jacques Polge, had a hit on his hands. **Coco** breaks new ground. It uses lots of flowers, but only as a purring, throbbing background. Jasmine, mimosa, rose, orange blossom and even frangipani are soft murmurs awash in a sea of amber spiked with clove bud, angelica and peach, with two big surprises yet to come. First there's the pungent assertiveness of leather notes, wild, burnished and bracing, then the final coup of real chocolate for that rich darkness that pervades **Coco**.

The total effect is, I think, more baroque than oriental; its husky tenacity and slight sweetness derive not from the stridency of eastern grasses, incenses and spices but from the opulent elegance of amber, leather and chocolate. It seems to breathe the air of exclusive salons, the luxurious comfort of well-established restaurants, the vivid electrics of opera. It is never at home when at home, demanding a much wider, more public arena in which to spread its cunning and seductive charms. **Coco** is not a kitten but a highly pedigreed cat. I always think of it as Colette prowling like a graceful, dangerous feline around the tables of the old Maxim's, claws drawn, smiling with mysterious mischief.

What to wear it with, where and when

Coco moves best in a world of red, black, amber, ivory, old gold, titian, tobacco, chocolate and stark black and white. It frowns disdainfully on pastels, blues and greens and it doesn't like much glitter either. Brunettes gravitate to it like a magnet, as do the titian and auburn-haired, but its intentions are too murky for a blonde. Clothes should be dramatic and simple, for day or night. Don't feature it too much in daylight (it can get especially cloying in heat) but let it radiate its warmth at night when you're out to impress or seduce. Definitely too dark and dangerous for the young, it is best worn by smart women who know exactly where they are going and with whom! Autumn and winter are its seasonal soul-mates, spring and summer being a touch too ingenuous for its calculated triumphs.

Cristalle
by Chanel

**PRONUNCIATION: kris-TARL
shar-NEL**

You may not have heard of this little known scintillation from Chanel, which has always stood in the shadows of its big sisters, **No. 5**, **No.19** and **Coco**. It's been there in the background since 1974, when it was introduced as a new form of perfume – almost an *extrait*, but not quite as strong. It was actually the forerunner of *eau de parfum*. But Chanel concentrated its publicity on its big guns, so poor **Cristalle** suffered somewhat from an identity problem. This neglect was recently rectified with a slight rearrangement of ingredients, aimed at pleasing the women who had grown up with it and now preferred a more 'modern' fragrance.

The new **Cristalle** is very charming, with an instantly sparkling appeal, and it keeps up that sparkle for quite some time. In the original, this was achieved by imbuing the middle notes with the same volatility of the top notes and then gradually revealing the base notes as a harmonic counterpoint. It now has a more citrusy charge, with high-pitched, crisp notes of mandarin and lemon softened by a persistent peach accord. Under this lies the heart of

Cristalle – a fetchingly arranged bouquet of honeysuckle, hyacinth, jasmine and roses, all bedded down with ylang ylang, amber, moss and gentle woods to give an autumnal haunting under the springtime freshness.

Cristalle's big secret is its unchanged harmony from beginning to finish. Its formulation is so artfully blended that there is a distinct but subtle progression from citrus to flowers to amber and wood, thus avoiding the monotonous, over-persistent single note of so many 'moderns' whose smell goes on and on and on, often to great annoyance. That alone makes it infinitely superior, and well worth discovering. **Cristalle** is quite a charmer in the Chanel tradition.

What to wear it with, where and when

While it may have brought a slightly older image upon itself with its reformulation, **Cristalle** still requires dressing that is essentially youthful and unfussy. For daywear it's quite comfortable in little suits and jackets with a tailored skirt, and sportswear of a superior cut. For evening it's not really in the grand league of extravaganzas but is perfectly poised in little cocktail dresses and evening suits with a dash of sparkle. Its colours tend toward the subdued sunnies – amber, copper, tobacco, mustard, curry, apricot, peach and cream, and it's not averse to black and white. **Cristalle** is best on those under forty, who will find that its fascinating sparkle moves from season to season with elegant ease.

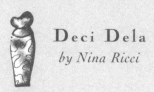

Deci Dela
by Nina Ricci

PRONUNCIATION: der-SEE der-LAH
NEEN-a REECH-ee

Somewhat frenetically described as a perfume for the woman who is 'here, there and everywhere', Ricci's very unconventional perfume hit the boulevards in 1994. Those expecting it to follow in the tradition of romantic **L'Air du Temps** were about to be surprised.

With an exuberant and saucy thumbing of the nose at the plethora of other fruit-based perfumes, **Deci Dela** shows its competitors that fruity perfumes don't necessarily have to dote on oranges, mandarins and nectarines. From its amphora-type bottle to its daring mixture of fruit, flowers and woods, this perfume sets out to create merry hell!

It begins its very extroverted enticement with peach, raspberry, red currant and watermelon – so luscious that the effect is quite salivating. Over this fruit salad comes the new 'headspace' technology (meaning very fresh, intense and lifelike) of osmanthus, a delicate apricot-scented Chinese blossom, and Australian boronia, with its sweet, wild and strong outdoorsy smell. Then come romantics like *rose de mai*, sweet pea and freesia, which underlines the boronia top note, attended by cedarwood, sandalwood, patchouli,

Sumatran balsam and the legendary Cambodian agarwood. Finally, there's a dark blaze of green with oakmoss, chypre resin and desert flower gums, and to cap it all off, a tropical flourish of deliciously ripe Javanese papaya!

Don't judge **Deci Dela** too hastily at first whiff. Let it relax and settle a couple of minutes and these notes will be gently transformed into a more luminous and soft *mélange* as the flowers and woods emerge. It's still a fairly punchy perfume, mind you, but its sparkle is absolutely infectious.

When perfumer Jean Guichard was given his brief from Ricci, he was asked to create something audacious but with 'even more' of everything. He gave them the works. Its 'even more' attitude is so witty, dynamic, whimsical and totally captivating, you'll wish you could drink its delicious sensuousness!

What to wear it with, where and when

Deci Dela is certainly not for the introvert. I don't think anyone over thirty should wear it unless they're still blessed with a gamine pertness. It is an absolute little devil on the young, though, coming on strong with vivacity and *joie de vivre*. It needs strong colours to complement its cheeriness — bright reds, oranges, yellows, gold. It also cuts quite a dash with white. Clothes should be clean-cut, even daring, in cotton, linen, silk, chiffon, tulle and denim (not necessarily blue). I think of it as a spring or summer sprite, day or night, and to be used quite lavishly; it's such a flirt you may as well let it have full rein.

Diorella
by Christian Dior

*I*n 1967 Dior unwittingly created what was to become almost a 'unisex' fragrance with the launch on the male market of **Eau Sauvage**. It was an instant hit with men, and women loved to smell its lemony freshness to such an extent they secretly bought or borrowed it for themselves, so the poor guys had yet another bastion of masculinity reefed out from under their jocks!

Maybe that's why, five years on, Dior created **Diorella**, a perfume specifically for women. While much more complex, fascinating and naturally more feminine than its male inspiration, the resemblance is startlingly obvious.

To create what is basically a citrus perfume that's attractive to women across a broad spectrum of tastes and behaviours is no mean feat, even for Dior. A purely citrus scent would tend to be too sharp, too penetrating and too masculine to attract the sophisticated woman. So, although it begins with a flood of boisterous Sicilian lemon and bergamot, **Diorella** very quickly (almost simultaneously) throws in armloads of sweet heady jasmine, honeysuckle and whispers of delicate hyacinth to smooth the biting edge, rounding it further with peach to give a delicious aureole.

Added to this is a scattering of green leaves, fern, oakmoss fixed with vetyver, and the merest hint of patchouli. It's all very subtle, but powerful enough to give **Diorella** a deliciously long life on the skin as it spins out its drifts of fragrance on the air.

There's never a doubt of its overall citrus theme, but the background of white flowers and greenery is ever-present, right through to the final lingering notes. A small masterpiece of harmony and balance, **Diorella** stands attractively apart from its enchanting sisters. It doesn't have the intense femininity of **Miss Dior**, the oriental mystique of **Dioressence**, the joyful innocence of **Diorissimo**, the voluptuousness of **Poison** or the enigmatic seascape of **Dune**. It is more like a sunny summer's day in the country – as golden yellow as van Gogh's sunflowers and as seemingly artless as a Matisse interior full of flowers and fruit. It's sparkling, shimmering, lilting and totally irresistible!

What to wear it with, where and when

Anything that smacks of a day in the country, or at least in the garden – yellow, green, white, azure, beige will suit perfectly. It needs bright, light clothes and is as great on the young as the more mature. Essentially a perfume for the day, it is also an invaluable travelling companion; one whiff of it banishes fatigue, jettisons jetlag and vaporises hefty hangovers! But don't expect it to be sensuous – it's far too light-hearted for heavy seductions.

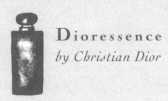

Dioressence
by Christian Dior

*M*en may have chuckled when Marlene Dietrich kicked off her high heels and followed Gary Cooper across the blazing Sahara in *Morocco*, but some women took an entirely different and empathetic view. After all, here was a beautiful, sophisticated and determined woman, ready to catch her man at all costs. She was a woman to be reckoned with!

There are plenty of women today of the same bent. Even though in these enlightened times they might jump into the four-wheel drive and drag him from the desert kicking and screaming, they are a definite breed unto themselves. They are definitely **Dioressence** women.

When Dior launched this oriental blockbuster in 1979, it took off in an entirely new direction from its stablemates. It headed, just like Marlene, straight for the beguiling mysteries and dangers of the Orient (or thereabouts). Its formulation broke new ground with its complex and challenging potpourri of flowers and spices generating a penetrating, pulsating warmth.

Based on cloves, cinnamon and patchouli with a generous dash of vanilla, **Dioressence** then adds the romantic softness of roses and jasmine with a hint of violet, a twist of citrus and a strong infusion of Spanish geranium – an essence not widely used in women's fragrances because of its pungent, pervasive tang. It's really the inclusion of geranium that sets **Dioressence** so singularly apart from its oriental rivals. It gives it a sharp dryness that is a perfect counterpoint to the lusty spices and flowers.

The woman who wears it with *élan* will be poised but with a wickedly humorous sense of devilry, a wily and understated seductiveness and *éclat* – just like our dear departed Marlene in her man-eating heyday. She may be all of that, but in the strong embrace of a Gary Cooper type she's all melting, submissive helplessness. **Dioressence** is like that!

What to wear it with, where and when

It has a distinct liking for lushly extravagant fabrics in gold, black, ruby, amber, topaz, copper, auburn, titian and moonstone colours. Don't bother with it by day; it's strictly nocturnal. Apart from dramatic swathes it adores the severe mannishness of tuxedos and pants, the svelteness of pyjama suits, kaftans, turbans, veils and masses of exotic jewellery. **Dioressence** is sensational in autumn and devastating in winter. If you're under twenty-five, however, you'll run the risk of being called all sorts of shady things, so save it for when you know the ropes!

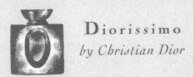

Diorissimo
by Christian Dior

S pring in a bottle, and all year round! Just a whiff of **Diorissimo** and you don't ever have to wait for those darling buds to bloom and blossom.

The great Christian Dior died in 1957, but a year before he commissioned a new fragrance that would epitomise his life-long love of the delicate and trembling *muguet*, or lily of the valley, as we know it. He stamped this beautiful motif on much of his creativity in the shape, line, colour and curve of his clothes.

Diorissimo was an instantaneous sensation. Parisian women in particular took it to their hearts and boudoirs, and very soon every woman of taste and elegance seemed to be awash in its joyous rapture. After a shortly respectable Gallic consideration, it was deemed a classic, an accolade almost unheard of in such a *jeune fille* perfume.

The first thing to say about **Diorissimo**, as far as liking it goes, is that if you personally don't care for the scent of lily of the valley then it will be absolute anathema to you. But if its light but intensely heady smell creates a delicious giddiness of the heart and spirit, you'll dote on **Diorissimo**. It's more than a single-flower fragrance, though, using other flowers to take the sharp edge off the main scent – like amaryllis lily, jasmine and a little ylang ylang. The perfume is also further softened with very light touches of amber and patchouli and a zing of fresh green leaves. Together they make **Diorissimo** unmistakably haunting.

Diorissimo is utterly disarming. It has the wonderful power of enveloping and flattering, of making you feel ecstatically happy when you weren't before. It is like receiving an unexpected gift of quivering, dew-dropped *muguet* fresh from the forest. If *that* doesn't disarm you, give the game away!

What to wear it with, where and when

Diorissimo was made for blondes, but is just as fetching on brunettes. Redheads may be a bit vivid for its pastel charms. If you're pushing thirty, forget it; leave it to the young, who deserve its rapturous overtures. It's an absolute knockout with all pinks, white, pale to bright greens and blues, lemon, lavender, mauve, violet, amethyst, cream, gold and silver. Clothes should be ultra-feminine, even a little fussy, and it's absolutely fabulous on brides (but not their mothers!). It blooms best on spring and summer afternoons and evenings. But be warned – **Diorissimo** is extremely youthful!

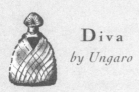

Diva
by Ungaro

PRONUNCIATION: DEEV-uh

oon-GAR-o

*I*t's tempting to liken **Diva** to an early Verdi opera – full to the brim with a bit of everything, and then some. A staggering array of ingredients exist in one big happy operatic ensemble, sometimes warbling in unison but more often than not singing to the audience, totally oblivious of others onstage! That's what makes **Diva** so fascinating – the way it keeps sending out surprise notes from its chorus of ingredients.

Your first encounter with this incendiary prima donna is likely to be thrilling, even a trifle unnerving. **Diva** does not suffer from stagefright; when the curtain goes up, it makes a grand entrance! The perfume first hit the boards in 1983, and it's very typical of its creator's *couture* style – highly complex, totally uncompromising and utterly unique.

Diva boasts a starry cast of Damascus and Moroccan roses, Mediterranean bergamot, iris, mandarin, narcissus, honey and oakmoss and, from the Far East, jasmine, ylang ylang, coriander, cardamom, vetyver, patchouli, rare woods and amber. It's this last ingredient that really steals the show, revealing itself at the finale with its deep base notes. Yet all this doesn't make **Diva** mysterious and impenetrable — anything but! Like a fine aria, it is by turns dazzling and demanding, with a brilliant cadenza of great virtuosity.

Ungaro reportedly created **Diva** for his muse, the ageless Anouk Aimée, and the perfume admirably catches her worldly-wise elegance and candour. But it reminds me more of Callas in mid-flight as Tosca, all unbridled passion and fabulous fury. And in key!

What to wear it with, where and when

To the opera, of course, and any other grand event. **Diva** is an indefatigable party goer and weaves an unabashedly seductive spell over dinner parties as well. Since it is far from innocent, prettiness in all forms must be avoided. Go for the dramatic, the devastating, the daring. Wear lots of gold and jewellery (the more baroque the better) and colours like burnished red, copper, amber, crimson, imperial purple and magenta. Black, silver and white are also fine. With its firebrand temperament, **Diva** is best at night, where it can unleash its operatic forces to standing ovation effect. The young had best wait in the wings, but to all other ages, **Diva** is a plum role. Seasons are immaterial to this prima donna — **Diva** will sing any time!

Dolce & Gabbana
by Dolce & Gabbana

PRONUNCIATION: DOL-cheh eh gab-ARNA

*I*f you're sick to death of high-powered, emphatic perfumes that seem to wear you instead of you wearing them, then breathe a sigh of relief, because Dolce & Gabbana, bless their sentimental Italian hearts, have created an almost absurdly old-fashioned perfume – but with a swish new twist.

Dolce & Gabbana is not so much a return to the refinement of the classics as much as a fetching and lovely extension of them. It doesn't boast anything enigmatic or sensational in its formulation; it is simply a gorgeously rich and sweet floral from which emerges a bracing exuberance of fruits, herbs, leaves and woods, all finished off with a sensuous drift of vanilla.

Its top note is jasmine, with lily of the valley and orange blossom in hefty support. These establish an engagingly feminine accord out of which comes the real zing: notes of cool ivy, the fascinating aniseed smell of basil and the just-picked tang of mandarin. It's this central note that persists as the fragrance progresses to the creamy depths of sandalwood, with a whiff of musk adding its haunting nostalgia.

Dolce & Gabbana is a very wearable perfume – versatile, undemonstrative, but sweepingly constructed to wrap you in an air of sensuousness. It's what you might call an elegant ally, and is a welcome respite from the rigours of those drop-dead dynamics of some other designer perfumes – which is probably why men twitch their noses with delight when **Dolce & Gabbana** wafts into their orbit!

What to wear it with, where and when

Its refined dazzle and panache make it provocative but always feminine, so clothes with an unconventional elegance are the go. They can be body clingers or sensuous and loose, even transparent if you like, but above all, light and sassy. **Dolce & Gabbana** loves sheeny fabrics, clothes with a thirties bias-cut look, unconventional casuals and dressed-up evening fripperies. It also slips easily into slinky suits and frothy little frou-frou numbers. Since it's a perfume full of life, it's great company at dinner parties (in fact, *any* party), gala occasions and cocktail bashes. Best of all, it doesn't care too much about age – twenty, thirty, forty-something it takes in its stride. However, older women might feel too frivolous in it. Wear it spring and summer, with lots of colour or basic shiny black, preferably with amusing jewellery or even a cute little hat for maximum impact. It's not a fragrance to be taken too seriously.

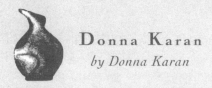

Donna Karan
by Donna Karan

PRONUNCIATION: DONN-uh ka-RAN

Just when you thought the rush of designer fragrances had safely passed, Donna Karan dived into the thick of things with her signature scent. Called simply **Donna Karan**, or **DK**, the perfume took its time getting to its expectant fans: Ms Karan had the perfume but not the presentation. But then her sculptor husband, Stephen Weiss, came up with a marvellous bottle design. It's quite a standout – a graceful but emphatic curve of moulded black with matt gold swipes as contrast. Very arresting, very dramatic. The contents can be described likewise.

Donna Karan is an intense, expressive blow to the senses right off. It possesses a warm strength that stops short of being overpowering as the perfume's structure cleverly unearths its complexities not in one all-conquering blast but in subtle gradations. Its revelations begin with vivacious top notes composed of exotic flowers – Casablanca lily, Moroccan jasmine, ylang ylang, rose, cassia, and the enigmatic but elegant heliotrope. These beauties are then wrapped in a lovely radiance of warm-hearted apricot, giving the calculated impression of a smooth, almost suede-like luxe. Then the darker, earthier notes infiltrate. Not content with being in the background, they quietly advance and arrange themselves around the lush bouquet. There's pungent patchouli, creamy sandalwood, golden amber, heady musk and, finally, a sensual veil of vanilla. As these gradations gather ranks, the perfume becomes more seductive and smouldering – like smoke trails in an autumnal forest. This gives it allusions to suede and cashmere – two textural favourites of Donna Karan.

This perfume has an air of belonging to you. It's an essential but invisible extension of a unique and highly individual style. Whether that style agrees with yours or not will determine whether you fall under its spell or shrug your shoulders at its Americanised orientalism.

What to wear it with, where and when

Being strictly a nocturnal animal, prowling, sleek and mysterious, **Donna Karan** was born for black. It's also a killer with navy and grey, dark reds and blues. If you're familiar with Donna Karan's style of dressing – cleverly understated, surprisingly dashing – then you know what to wear with it. **Donna Karan** adores social gatherings of a rather chatty, jazzy tone and is charming if not too liberally applied over dinner. Keep it away from the office; although it's not an outright seducer, it might come in for bitchy comment. This is very much an autumn and winter perfume, and if you're under thirty, forget it!

Donna Trussardi
by Trussardi

PRONUNCIATION: troo-SARR-dee

I hope this recent addition to the prestigious stable of Trussardi doesn't suffer a similar fate to its august predecessor, **Trussardi**. That fabulously original perfume, stunningly encased in a white leather flask, was not everyone's idea of perfume with its rich, woody individualism, but *aficionados* have long since treated it as a treasure. Sweet little sister **Donna** has a hard act to follow, but she makes the grade with the younger market with her winning ways and heart-on-the-sleeve enthusiasm. She charmed the judges of the English *New Woman* magazine Beauty Awards in 1994, picking up a commendation for Best New Fragrance. Not a bad start!

Donna Trussardi can be roughly categorised as a chypre-floral but with the accent on flowers underpinned by spices and herbs. In structure it's not unlike the lovely **Miss Dior**, but definitely younger and more innocent, although the rumblings of sensuality can be detected just below the surface. **Donna Trussardi** has a most infectious sparkle. It opens with a wonderful rush of heady jasmine and sweet, lingering hyacinth, infused with strong dashes of cardamom, coriander and ginger, and more than a hint of violet. This delicious accord is then heightened with the snap of tangerine and the dark brilliance of blackcurrant. Out of all this excitement, a calm centre of Turkish rose, ylang ylang, iris and lily of the valley slowly emerges, accompanied by patchouli, sandalwood, juniper and some musk-tinged ambrette. But long after you've applied **Donna Trussardi** you'll be left with a strong impression of coriander, ginger and cardamom synthesised with violet and hyacinth.

This is a rich and romantic, but not sentimental, perfume. It has no grand seductions in mind, but is nevertheless totally disarming. A charming and irresistible flirt, **Donna Trussardi** is very easy to fall for.

What to wear it with, where and when

If you're a little too mature for frills, flounces, bows, tiny boleros and low-slung jeans, then **Donna Trussardi** is not for you. Nobody over thirty has a hope of carrying it off, but those under this age will have a giddy, dizzy time playing up to its light-hearted caprices. It's great with all vibrant colours, pastels and plenty of white, but steer clear of neutrals, heavies and black. It's quite at home day or night, so you can slip out of your jeans into a saucy little cocktail frou-frou with it still enveloping you sweetly. **Donna Trussardi** loves having a great time wherever she goes, and that's just about everywhere! Best in the warmer months, it is a little too reckless for winter.

Dune
by Christian Dior

Dune follows in the controversial footsteps of the previous two Dior fragrances, **Poison** for women and **Fahrenheit** for men, throwing away like its predecessors the safety net of having the name 'Dior' in its title. When in 1992 it emerged Venus-like from the sea of perfumes already threatening to drown us, **Dune** swept its competition aside in one brilliant fell swoop.

Definitely not related to the sands of the Sahara but rather to the wilder, sweeter shores of deserted beaches and thundering surf, **Dune** is a unique perfume, one which has created its own category. Dior confidently called it 'the first floral-oceanic', which is a fair enough boast, I suppose. It certainly isn't a floral in the ordinary sense. If anything it veers toward the dry, spicy, woody category that dominates the male end of the fragrance market. Indeed, at first smell I thought it smelt primarily masculine – a misconception that soon was dispelled as it opened its heart and soul.

Specifically, **Dune** contains such esoteric components as lichen, broom, the sweet-scented wallflower, the majestic peony and warm, resinous amber. All this adds up to a windswept sweetness and a certain sunset glow. It's one of those rebel smells that is totally uncompromising, that takes you by surprise but remains doggedly mysterious.

Don't underestimate its strength – it's very tenacious, so be relatively sparing lest it comes on like a tidal wave! Once it settles on the skin it exudes its atmospherics of the beach and the sea, elevating the senses and sending a rush of childhood nostalgia through you.

In its softly curved bottle and pale coral packaging, **Dune** is something of an enigma. However, its credentials are so well bred as to assure it a place among the soon-to-be classics. It's certainly engendered much opinion, both for and against. I'm definitely for it, but I shudder at the thought of the ineptitiude of its inevitable imitators. May a sudden sandstorm sweep them all out to sea to their deservedly watery graves!

What to wear it with, where and when

Dune is a sunny number, outdoorsy and extroverted. This being the case, its only liking for the grand occasion is to appear in great drifts of chiffon, untold yards of organza, lamé and lace, all designed very simply and in sand or sea colours – never anything as blatant as purple or red, although gold and silver are fine. It's no good at all with black or grey, needing warm, honeyed tones to bring out its mysterious individuality. **Dune** is snappy with smart daywear, be it at the office or out shopping, and is at ease at cocktail bashes and the like. The young can get away with it, although it's at its mature best with the twenty to forty age bracket.

Eden
by Cacharel

PRONUNCIATION: cash-a-REL

*I*t's been a long time between inspirations at Cacharel since the introduction of **Loulou** in 1987 and **Anaïs Anaïs** a while before that. But with **Eden**, Cacharel restates its commitment to perfumes with definite appeal to younger women. With this in mind, **Eden** veers away from the innocence of **Anaïs Anaïs** and the sensuality of **Loulou** into an altogether different territory. It's even invented a new subcategory for itself called 'wet floral oriental', which means it uses aquatic plants as well as sweet earthy ones and adds a dash of spices to balance.

To begin with we have waterlilies, lotus flowers and the delicacy of rushflowers. That's the aquatic team. Then comes a lovely whiff of watermelon and pineapple given more deliciousness with hypnotic orange blossom, mimosa (the European counterpart of acacia) and patchouli grass. Add a tang of leafy greenery and the harmonic chord is complete. You will find, however, that a luscious fruity smell filters through to be the dominant, but never domineering, influence. This is not the Garden of Eden and all its drama between Adam, Eve and the Serpent, but a more serene earthly paradise. And I think that's why the perfume succeeds.

Eden is quite elusive at first whiff and you may feel a little disappointed. But leave it to develop on your skin a while and its enchantment will slowly reveal itself with a soft fruitiness counterbalanced by an insistent undercurrent of haunting flowers not often found in other perfumes.

The sense of innocence not yet lost is symbolised in **Eden**'s beautiful, marbled jade asymmetrical bottle, all coolness and tranquillity. This is the outer summation of a perfume I think is exquisite for its peaceful, understated subtlety and youthful charm.

What to wear it with, where and when

Although obviously aimed at the young woman, **Eden** is not out of the orbit of the more mature. I think it's one of those rare perfumes that crosses so-called age barriers, so it will smell as fetching on a teenager as on an eighty-year-old. All it really requires is that the wearer be lighthearted and outgoing. Don't wear dark colours with it. **Eden** suits clear, light colours like blue, green, pink, yellow and cream. Black is off limits, and so is too much glitter. Clothes should be simple day or evening affairs of cotton, linen, georgette, chiffon or silk. It's more at home in spring and summer, especially in the afternoon and early evening, when it exudes its endearing young charms with a soft insistence.

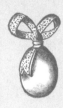

Elizabeth Taylor's
Diamond Collection:

WHITE DIAMONDS
DIAMONDS & EMERALDS
DIAMONDS & RUBIES
DIAMONDS & SAPPHIRES

*A*fter unleashing her unbridled **Passion** on us some time ago, the lovely Elizabeth turned to her second weapon, diamonds, as the inspiration for her follow-up perfume.

Whoever created **White Diamonds** came amazingly close to capturing the diamond's icy incandescence. **White Diamonds** is brilliant, high-pitched and crackling with zing. Based on white flowers of the outspoken variety – mainly tuberose and narcissus – the perfume is kept under control with the soft and haunting scent of the Amazon lily. The luminosity of these flowers is given a velvet touch with seductive oakmoss and a hint of patchouli for a faraway mystique that's most intriguing and suggestive. **White Diamonds** turns heads without swivelling them; it makes its presence felt with an effervescent insistence.

Its success naturally led to a set of variations on the theme – diamonds with emeralds, rubies and sapphires. **Diamonds & Emeralds** is richly verdant with lashings of gardenia underlined with something piquant that smells like green tea. The effect is surprisingly al fresco, like a lush bouquet that lingers long on the evening air. It's a fragrance that wears its heart on its silken sleeve.

Diamonds & Rubies, on the other hand, is all roses and mystery. It has a hypnotic depth given an intriguing twist with a touch of tuberose and a faintly spicy smell like carnations. It is sweet, seductive and utterly romantic.

The last perfume in Miss Taylor's quartet, **Diamonds & Sapphires**, sends off sharp sparks of full-blown, heady jasmine – lingering, lilting and luxurious, with tantalising undertones of delicious ripe fruits. Its approach is slightly more youthful than its sisters, less serious, more flirtatious.

All four are presented with typical Hollywood gorgeousness in teardrop globes nestling in velvet-lined boxes, each topped with a glittering *faux* diamond bow set with the appropriate coloured stones. When presented with one or all, a woman will imagine herself caught in the giddy spin of Liz-type luxury. Well, after all, anyone can dream . . .

What to wear them with, where and when

The clues here are obvious – it's glamour and sparkle all the way. There's not much use featuring one of these darlings dressed in a cotton frock on a picnic! All of the **Diamonds** thrive on the Big Occasion. You'll need to be fittingly seductive, or at least sensuous, but definitely not vulgar (Miss Taylor is *always* the lady). Don't bother with these perfumes in broad daylight; keep them until the cocktail hour and any time thereafter, depending on what plans are afoot. They sparkle beautifully in any season.

Escape
by Calvin Klein

*T*he directive from on high was to create 'something fresh but not green – with an ozonic note, but not salty; essentially something outdoors but sensuous'. And with Calvin Klein already having decided on the name, it was perfumer Ann Gottlieb who came up with the goods for him.

Escape is the operative word in many ways – an escape back to nature, escape from the stress of modern living, escape into one's inner sanctum of private pleasures. Although one of the new 'ozonic' perfumes – a child of Dior's great **Dune** – it sticks close to the land with its medley of fruits and flowers over spices, grasses and wood. The open-air motif which dominates is achieved by a cleverly balanced accord of hyacinth, lily of the valley and osmanthus, plus a mouth-watering dash of lychee. To bolster this light-headed aura, a touch of nostalgic mandarin, apple, blackcurrant, plum and peach are added. And to make sure the concoction doesn't disappear into the upper air, dashes of Indian vetyver grass, a wraith of clove-like spice, a golden glow of marigold, a veil of musk, and tonka beans with a smooth overlay of sensuously dry sandalwood firm and round the whole thing into a fascinating and not-too-tenacious synthesis.

Escape is an exhilarating perfume that can either take you away or make sure you have a lovely time if you are already there. It's not so much an escape route but a safe arrival and a happy time in the never-never.

What to wear it with, where and when

Escape is a holiday companion, whether you're on one on not. It revels in dressed-down clothes of the superbly cut kind. Everything must be light and airy: no fancy fabrics, no heavy or vibrant colours. It's much more relaxed in pastels, neutrals and white. It reels away from the sombreness of black and grey, and is strictly a spring and summer relaxer. Age doesn't matter a hoot, so it's an ideal fragrance to give as a gift. Even if you can't take it dearly to your own heart, **Escape** is one of those stand-by reliables for when the black moods attack you and you want to get away from it all. Simply use it as your escape hatch!

Estée
by Estée Lauder

*T*his Lauder luminary invites you to wear it and 'create your own fantasy' – a pretty presumption that could lead to all sorts of extraordinary things.

Of all the Lauder fragrances **Estée** is certainly the most enigmatic and difficult to pin down. It actually smells mighty like a moss rose – a rose you have to get right into the heart of to catch its world of private and guarded exquisiteness. Once in its clutches it completely captivates you.

Although originally touted as 'the first superperfume' and noted for its long-lasting potency, **Estée** is anything but demanding. It is definite but refined, appealing to the modern woman of worldly sophistication and self-confidence, rather like its sister oriental **Cinnabar**.

Estée has an exultant top note of Moroccan rose absolute and complex harmonies provided by tuberose, jasmine and lily of the valley. To add dash and spice there's a good solid whack of carnation. But the two big surprises that give it its sense of mystical adventure are the intense herbiness of Russian coriander and the foresty elusiveness of Balkan tree moss. It's these two green, woody and mossy catalysts that carry the rose to a more elevated, imperious position and also trigger the other flowers into pulsating action. It's a very inventive idea and one that works to give the perfume its rather aloof stance of individuality.

Estée entices you to journey far from the madding crowd, your destination unplanned, your mind open to new experiences and ready to accept the upshot. This, I suppose, qualifies it as a fantasy perfume. So, if you're the type, Estée is just the ticket to take you who-knows-where.

What to wear it with, where and when

Estée is extremely elegant, so only the best will pass muster. Quietly rich colours and clothes are most suited to its refined approach – lovely cream silk or georgette tea gowns, ice-blue satin evening dresses. Of course you can add a touch of individualistic fantasy, but certainly nothing showy. Estée moves in privileged circles with innate poise and confidence, so that precludes the young (who wouldn't be attracted to its subtleties anyway). But it's wonderful on young-mature and older women. Essentially an afternoon and evening perfume for spring and summer, it's absolutely perfect to wear to the likes of a chamber music recital or to waft around in looking at a new art exhibition.

Eternity
by Calvin Klein

'**R**omance with commitment. That's what today's woman wants.' So saith Calvin Klein in describing the inspiration for this lovely perfume. After the raunchiness of **Obsession**, **Eternity** comes like peace after the holocaust, and it arrives fully equipped with romantic trappings as promised, but romance of the new-age, unsentimental sort.

There's certainly nothing pretty or dainty about **Eternity**. It doesn't wear its heart on its sleeve; more like under its shoulder pads. It attempts to redefine in perfumed terms the contemporary stance on romance: no frills, no glitter, but kind-hearted commonsense instead – an intelligent approach to matters of the heart based on equality and trust rather than swooning passions.

All of which means there's nothing terribly complex or cunning about **Eternity**. It melds together a quartet of sweet-scented white flowers against a balanced background of fruits and woods. Freesia, lily, lily of the valley and narcissus are fused into a strong floral phalanx brought up in the rear by mandarin and sandalwood. Also present are rare wildflowers and patchouli, which are kept behind the frontline attack. It all adds up to a perfume that stays doggedly faithful to its initial impact from go to whoa.

Eternity is a relatively soft and penetrating perfume. It has a bright cleanness that's a welcome change from the brash brigade, and it deserves its devoted following. Yet, despite all this, I find it a curiously old-fashioned smell: it is an ardent perfume that is determined to please.

Perhaps its very inoffensiveness is its limitation. Then again, the neo-romantics for whom it was designed are not complaining.

What to wear it with, where and when

If you're remotely familiar with the Calvin Klein look in clothes then you'll get the **Eternity** message right off. If it's clean, almost severe, and preferably white or neutral in colour, then you're on the right track. I'm not particularly mad about its being worn in the evening — I think it's much better suited to afternoons. It's a good hostess fragrance, giving you a fresh, polished and poised aura. **Eternity** is not for the very young or the very mature, but perfect for the middle age bracket, when a woman is either up for grabs or has grabbed it and wants to keep the flame alive for as long as possible. I don't think it's very suited to winter, but if you're fleeing the cold, take it on holidays with you to warmer climes. It's a pleasant travelling companion.

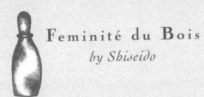

Feminité du Bois
by Shiseido

PRONUNCIATION: fam-IN-itay doo-BWAR she-SHADE-o

When, a few years ago, this Japanese-based house opened a sumptuously austere new *parfumerie* in *Les Salons de Palais Royal,* its new resident genius, Serge Lutens, created this astonishingly original perfume for the much-publicised event.

Feminité du Bois was Lutens's beloved child, inspired by walks around the exotic, mysterious streets near his home in Marrakesh. Here, apart from the indigenous fragrances of Morocco, the air is permeated with the unmistakable smell of cedar from the Atlas Mountains nearby. The scent of cedarwood and cedar oil is insistent and soft, but has a considerable tenacity. Using very high concentrations of cedar as all three dominating notes in the top, middle and base of his perfume, Lutens began to add other, surprisingly harmonic, notes: Moroccan rose for sweetness, cardamom for intense spiciness, peach for mellowness, honey for warmth and smoothness, and musk for an underlying sensuality that also serves to fix this magic potion. For Lutens it was an audacious adventure into fascinating, untrodden regions of scent.

Lutens envisioned a perfume so sensual it would be almost animalistic. In this he succeeded most admirably. **Feminité du Bois** is sinuous and insidious. It floats a veil of calm repose over you, then gradually unfurls its erotic tentacles to completely capture you in a hypnotic daze. Arrestingly packaged in a curved phial of deep plum opaque glass designed to be symbolic of a female form in repose, it reflects the Lutens fascination with light, shape and colour. **Feminité du Bois** is audaciously assertive yet as maddeningly elusive as a purple Moroccan night. You don't so much put it on as surrender yourself to it.

What to wear it with, where and when

If it's soft and sensuous, wear it — especially if it's dreamy blue, pale rose, dusky pink, cloudy amethyst, frosted heliotrope, pearl grey, peach or cream. This perfume is all langour and laziness. Keep it for late afternoons, mysterious twilights, intimate evenings — it's not a crowd pleaser or a party stopper. **Feminité du Bois** is ageless and seasonless, a fine companion when you need the salve of tranquillity.

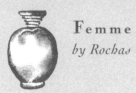

Femme
by Rochas

PRONUNCIATION: FAM
hro-SHAR

*T*here's *un petit mystère* about the introduction of this perfume that's typically French. One source has it that Marcel Rochas sent a letter to a select group of women in 1944 offering them his new, limited-edition *parfum*. Because they adored it, he made it available to women at large. Another source maintains that Rochas had the perfume specifically created for his bride-to-be. Madame Rochas could be forgiven for thinking her husband was an Indian-giver when suddenly it was no longer hers alone, but available to anyone with the money to buy it!

Anyhow, whichever version is true, the upshot of it all was that **Femme** became a roaring success and has stayed the distance to this day. Although it did undergo a 'reorchestration' in 1989, the 'new' **Femme** smells about the same to me. It is still as beautiful, radiant and warmly embracing as ever, and remains the quintessential classic of the fruity-flowery category. The first deep sniff of it establishes its individuality. It smells of ripe, juicy, sun-warmed fruit from a French orchard – peaches, plums, apples, pears, apricots and citrus fruits – all married to very elegant flowers, chiefly jasmine and roses. Added to this is a soft roundelay of green chypre notes, very controlled and without any sharpness to mar the hush of everything, together with dark, velvety oakmoss and dashes of patchouli, amber and musk to round out the mellow harmonies.

All of this gives **Femme** a delicious, almost salivating sensuality. It is a truly ravishing perfume, giving out sunny glints through the full-fruited orchard suspended in misty dusk. And in its amphora-curved, graceful bottle and its black Chantilly lace packaging, it's as beautiful to look at as it is to experience. In many ways, **Femme** is true to its name. It manages quite effortlessly to epitomise woman with all her moods, mysteries, wiles and charms.

What to wear it with, where and when

The key word here is 'rich' – rich fabrics, rich colours, rich clothes. Beautiful silks, wools, satins, brocades, velvets, chiffons, laces and lamés in the colours of the earth and orchard are ideal. To wear **Femme**, it's almost mandatory to be over twenty-five, and if you're pushing ninety you'll still exude a gentle loveliness. It's absolutely glorious in autumn and winter, and vibrant in spring and summer. No sophisticated woman should ever run out of it.

Fendi
by Fendi

PRONUNCIATION: FEN-dee

I first tried **Fendi** in Bali: a grave mistake. It got such a shock the perfume fainted dead away. It just didn't agree with the alien heat. But, be that as it may, **Fendi** is torrid enough to generate its own warmth, especially in considerably cooler climes.

This perfume was created by the eight Fendi sisters, renowned in the fashion industry for their witty and whimsical use of fur and leather. The stamp of unbridled Roman brio is ultimately the Fendi signature (or signatures), so when the redoubtable eight got together as a collective 'nose' to formulate ideas for their first perfume, it was bound to turn out a fragrant interpretation of Rome in all its splendour, past and present. And splendid it is!

Although an elusive little scamp to begin with, **Fendi** is complex enough to take its own time, little by little revealing its neoclassical dimensions. Taking the classic rose and jasmine alliance in quite powerful concentration, it deliberately overlays it with a head-on, passionate explosion of patchouli and ylang ylang – two forces to be reckoned with. But this eclipse works, especially when soft sandalwood, musk, amber and iris are added to round out and faintly blur the dramatics. Then, after theatrical dashes of spice and sharp citrus oils, and a slight greening with chypre, comes an audacious addition: leather. This ingredient, fashionable in perfumes of the twenties and thirties, has been largely ignored since, but a return to its animalic and burnished polish is a most imaginative and, in the case of **Fendi**, almost an in-house inevitability.

The entire creation has a Romanesque flamboyance of great sensuality and dash. **Fendi** has that typical Roman enthusiasm for life – like Anna Magnani in her more passionate moods. It may seem a little off-key in Bali, but in Rome it's a thrilling though elegant celebration of *la dolce vita*!

What to wear it with, where and when

In autumn and winter **Fendi** is a natural with rich colours like topaz, ginger, copper and gold, and it loves creamy ivory as well. Black is second nature to it, as well as rich browns. Clothes should be dramatic and unequivocal. Being of the Fendi clan, it was born to extravagant furs, leathers, suedes and velvets. It also adores animal prints, especially leopard and crocodile, and is a knockout with cashmere, mohair and alpaca. **Fendi** works better on brunettes and redheads than blondes, on fine olive skins rather than the peaches-and-cream brigade. Wear it to important parties, first nights and fabulous banquets, but not to Bali!

Ferre
by Gianfranco Ferre

PRONUNCIATION: fair-AI(R)
jarn-FRUNK-o

One look at the dynamic packaging of this stunner and you know you'll be thrown into the deep end. This is no lustrous white-flower virgin like Ferre's earlier signature perfume, **Gianfranco Ferre**; this is a troublemaker, a sharp-shooter, a cat among the pigeons.

The bottle looks disturbingly like a black bomb, its gold top dangerously resembling a hand grenade pin. But the blow is somewhat softened by its encasement in a black silk net, giving it a *femme fatale* seduction.

Ferre is dazzling, sensual, exotic and explosive. It's not so much the principal ingredients that give it its sizzle, it's the concentrations of them. Unstopper the bottle and you're hit with a powerful profusion of orange blossom and bergamot – a heady duo redolent of an orchard at blazing noon. Once exposed, this volatile mixture detonates an extremely strong and alluring battery of big floral scents – mainly rose and iris, the latter giving a sharp violet presence urging the most out of the roses. Over this is laid the pervasive lusciousness of ripe, warm peach and exotic passionfruit. The stage is set for fireworks – a display of perfume pyrotechnics that seems to go on firing fusilades for an extraordinarily long time.

Ferre has a tenacity that is so expertly balanced it never palls or fades to staleness. It has the remarkable quality of receding gradually while beckoning to follow. Italian in its stance, it unashamedly comes on with guns blazing in a torrent of bravado and relentless seduction. Like Ferre's spectacular creative takeover of the Dior fashion collections, it is almost excessive in its extravagance, but it has the clout to remain brilliant, electric and undeniably devastating. Handled with care, it guarantees a sure-fire hit at a helpless target!

What to wear it with, where and when

Ferre needs clothes with dash, pizzazz and swagger. Like Ferre's *couture*, it's made for worldly, rich and extravagant women with a taste for seduction and extroversion. Don't bother with charming little dresses, pert suits, floating fantasies or neutral casuals. Ferre has class, and so must you! Colours don't matter, as long as they're definite, and fabrics must reek of luxe – fabulous silks, leather, brocades, taffetas and furs. Ferre is for the mature and fearlessly self-confident woman only. Wear it to occasions rather than *tête-à-têtes*, but save it for evenings only, and expect fireworks! Don't worry about seasons – it sizzles all year round.

Fidji
by Guy Laroche

*A*nother plump mango plops to the ground, followed by a big green coconut, while you languish in a rope hammock threading frangipanis and hibiscus flowers into a lei. That just about sums up this sumptuously delicious perfume.

When Laroche launched **Fidji** in 1966, he sailed a perfumed voyage to the fabled tropical isles of the Pacific. As one of the very first adventures in perfume to combine a number of very powerful floral notes with an equally powerful profusion of green tonalities, **Fidji** remains unique. It's one of the most beautiful, compelling and downright friendly perfumes I know of. Though it's dreadfully underrated, probably because it's been around a while, **Fidji** speaks its own language of loveliness.

Its hugely extravagant bouquet of Florentine iris, French carnation, Egyptian tuberose, Bulgarian rose, Madagascan ylang ylang, Moroccan orange blossom and Italian jasmine forms a heady cascade layered with softly murmuring sandal and cedar woods, Malaysian patchouli, Persian musk, amber and Arabian balsam. All this is topped with vivid green notes of Spanish galbanum and Indian myrrh and vetyver. There may even be some English lilac lurking amongst all this too!

Strangely enough, this united nations conglomeration results in a smell you wouldn't expect – one that evokes but doesn't actually contain tropical blockbusters like frangipani, gardenia, ginger blossom, mango and guava. There's no holding back with **Fidji**. It was not meant to be refined or discreet, but it certainly stops (just!) this side of being vulgar. In fact, **Fidji** is so delicious you almost feel you want to drink it. Just make sure you've got that flaming red hibiscus behind the appropriate ear when you spray on its hypnotic lusciousness.

What to wear it with, where and when

It's a knockout with anything bright, tropical, jungle-like or flamboyant. Whatever you wear, keep it to a minimum; **Fidji** doesn't like fuss or frills. Age doesn't matter a jot as long as you look the part and are ready to let those sexy trade winds blow through your hair and the white moonlit sand squelch up through your toes. This perfume's not much cheer in autumn and winter, but come spring you'll be reaching for its exotic magic.

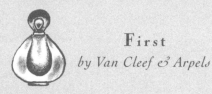

First

by Van Cleef & Arpels

This extraordinary perfume can claim the right to its lofty name for two reasons. For starters, it was the first perfume to be created by this grand French jewellery house, and secondly, it is reputed to be the first perfume to use (and, what's more, use lavishly) a most extraordinary ingredient in its complex formulation – the humble blackcurrant.

Of course, fruits have been used in perfume from time immemorial, and some modern perfumes have proved triumphs of their use – like Rochas's **Femme** and Dior's **Diorella**, to name but two. But blackcurrant doesn't seem to have been in the running until its revolutionary use in 1976 in the formula of **First**.

The perfume contains a number of other remarkable ingredients too. First, there's rose – not just any old rose, but the heavy, musky exotics of Turkish rose. Then there's the extraordinarily powerful scent of Italian jasmine and the rare and precious ylang ylang flower from the Cormorant Isles. Sandalwood, oakmoss, patchouli, vetyver, tonka bean, mandarin and narcissus leaves come next, followed by the lurking thrill of tuberose and the *pièce de résistance* of blackcurrant buds. Wed all this to the seductions of musk and amber, and you have a highly potent recipe for success.

This is not a 'nice' fragrance; this is a powerhouse perfume! The dazzle it detonates is instantly incandescent and thrilling, haunting you long after the initial shock. Don't be scared of **First**; beneath its dynamism it's surprisingly dignified. It is challenging, but the woman who realises its clever tactics and how to play into its hands will treasure it and treat it with the respect she would a precious jewel.

What to wear it with, where and when

First is the domain of the worldly, highly sophisticated and cultivated woman. It also belongs to the strategist – the seducer who wants to appear to be seduced. It's way out of line on the young, the reticent and the timid. If you can't wear black velvet head to toe, forget **First**! It's definitely a night-owl prowler, daylight being too gauche for its sauveness. And it's not an at-home perfume either; it has to be out and about, and to all the very best places. Apart from black it loves the dark, rich colours – never anything paler than purple, except rich cream. It demands fur, leather, suede, brocade, heavy silk in sweeping dresses and lots of fabulous jewellery to go with its haughty heritage. **First** blazes warmly through autumn and winter, but gets too aloof in the lighter seasons.

Fleur d'interdit
by Givenchy

PRONUNCIATION: fler dan-ter-DEE
zjhiv-on-SHE

What a wonderful influence Audrey Hepburn and Hubert de Givenchy had upon each other. It was as long ago as 1957 that Givenchy created a perfume exclusively for the lovely actress – a glorious gamine called **L'interdit**. When it was eventually released at large, it enjoyed a breathless popularity.

Now, years later, Givenchy pays tribute to his muse once again with this marvellously light and lovely fragrance. Although **Fleur d'interdit** doesn't have the spicy, mischievous kick of its mentor-perfume, it still has a brilliantly fresh outlook on life, love, and especially youth.

It begins its subtle persuasion with a trio of luscious fruits – raspberry, melon and peach. This is followed by a wonderful floral tapestry of rose, cyclamen, lilac, lily of the valley and violet leaf interwoven with a hint of gardenia. These ingredients are then combined with the dryness of sunflower and sandalwood and given a dash of vanilla. The gentle harmony of all these ingredients is achieved as if by osmosis – and that's why **Fleur d'interdit** has that signature synergy, the Givenchy trademark of elegance.

Like his *couture*, nothing is allowed to dominate; everything is there for a purpose.

The charm of the perfume (it comes only as *eau de parfum* or *cologne,* but is nevertheless strong enough to make its presence felt) is summated by its pretty pink and pale green packaging, the rose pink perfume itself in a frosted glass bottle with a simple gold ring around its neck. No *jeune fille* could fail to resist it – and nor should she. To wear a Givenchy with Hepburn associations couldn't fail to achieve a sense of romantic but light-hearted panache!

What to wear it with, where and when

Fleur d'interdit is made for pastels – the whole pretty lot of them, from lavender to lemon. It's a nosegay, a *fête* of nature in spring mood, and the clothes to be worn with it are simple, flowing, romantic and giddy. Hats, large and small, scarves, floaty overshirts, pretty blouses and swishy evening dresses are all lovely with its delicate persuasions. It's just as carefree and enchanting outdoors as well as in. It's impossible to imagine any women over thirty wearing **Fleur d'interdit**. As a fragrance that's almost impossible to overdo, it's a lovely introduction to the grown-up world of perfume for emerging butterflies. Wear it in spring and summer only – it's far too softly spoken and whimsical for colder weather.

Gianfranco Ferre
by Gianfranco Ferre

PRONUNCIATION: jarn-FRUNK-o fair-AI(R)

*C*s the wildly beautiful Claudia Cardinale glides into the arms of the madly handsome Alain Delon in the mesmerising ball scene from Visconti's *The Leopard*, one imagines her leaving an entrancing trail of Ferre's eponymous perfume in her whirling crinoline wake.

I don't think there's any more devastatingly beautiful, deliciously pervasive or frustratingly evasive perfume in the world today. I assume the perfume was created before Ferre took over the creative reigns at Christian Dior, since not only does **Gianfranco Ferre** have nothing to do with Dior, it doesn't have much to do with France either, being a typically full-blown romantic Italian enchantment. It's as if the white-flowering garden of a grand *palazzo* had drifted indoors, infiltrating lush late-Baroque interiors with its hypnotic grace and charm.

In composition it's an extraordinarily rich perfume, with a profusion of flowers infused with musk as a sensuous anchor to its sweetly discreet pleasures. Jasmine and lily of the valley begin the spell, along with tuberose, freesia and honeysuckle. This magical *mélange* is then poised over tender clove buds, green leaves, vetyver and sandalwood, all rounded off with musk used with a sparing hand. In all, it's a stunningly lovely collage – a perfume definitely of the garden, not the hothouse, variety.

I think of **Gianfranco Ferre** as a nocturnal perfume because of its elegant, romantic poignancy, its softly sensuous invitation. It is an utterly beguiling and persuasive scent which deserves greater popularity than it enjoys. It is not a hugely strong perfume, but is tenacious enough without being interfering. It may disappear quickly on some skins, but if that's so, simply put it on cottonwool pads tucked away at various vantage points – anywhere it can keep transmitting its subtle but delicious message. You won't have to wear a crinoline or have a handsome man on your arm; it will transmit its beautiful, romantic image even if you're alone – which you won't be for long!

What to wear it with, where and when

Romance is the word! Wear it with lashings of lace, chiffon, silk, brocade, satin, organza, tulle – all the filmy, floaty fabrics, in white, pastels, and any other softly feminine colours. No frills are necessary – simple drifts will do. Age is of little importance, but the right temperament is vital: you must be beguiling, elegant, poised and flirty, so viragos shouldn't bother! Spring and summer are best, especially languid afternoons and bewitching twilights. **Gianfranco Ferre** is a perfume that's absolutely wonderful to be wooed in; chaps go weak at the knees faced with its delicate seduction.

Gianni Versace
V'E
Versus Donna
by Gianni Versace

PRONUNCIATIONS:

ji-AHN-ee verrr-SART-chee

vee-EE

ver-suz DON-uh

I'm treating these as a trio, not because they're inseparable, but because they share a common Versace theme. What's more, the smart woman could very well use them as the basis of her perfume wardrobe.

The signature perfume, **Gianni Versace**, appeared in 1982. The second, **V'E**, appeared seven years later, and the third, **Versus Donna**, burst upon a hectic perfume scene in 1992 after the phenomenal success of **Versus** for men.

Versace's three babies have their head in clouds of myrrh, musk, incense, patchouli, amber and sandalwood. But it's what goes over the top of this exotica that gives each perfume its distinct personalitiy.

Gianni Versace is a super-rich formulation with layer upon layer of flowers: jonquil, honeysuckle, tuberose, orange flower, French marigold, jasmine, lavender and ylang ylang. This immense profusion is floated over warm chords of oakmoss and broom, plus an aromatic resin called olibanum.

Then come the Versace fleshpots of amber, patchouli, musk and sandalwood. The effect is thrilling, the impact enormous.

With this perfume, only the most dazzling clothes should be worn – in colours to match! It's fine for the afternoon but really rises to after-dark social occasions. The woman who wears **Gianni Versace** is nobody's fool.

V'E, on the other hand, is very light-hearted and vivacious, with loads of lovely big lilies and trembling lilies of the valley. These are joined by white hyacinth, jonquil, a touch of bergamot and green leaves to give a bracing freshness and to hold the immediacy of the flowers. This pretty posy is then given the classic depth of Bulgarian rose, jasmine, Florentine iris and ylang ylang before the Versace exotics take hold, allowing the flowers to trumpet out a collective fanfare. You won't mistake V'E.

It should be featured with anything clever, head-turning or just plain silly. It adores parties, discos, loud restaurants and dangerous living, so the older set is not in the race.

The youngest of the Versace sisters, **Versus Donna**, is full of surprising ingredients, beginning with blackcurrant, raspberry and plum. Then the floral tributes pour in: heliotrope, boronia, tuberose and black roses. These are followed by the Versace coup of musk and amber with a dash of iris and sandalwood. Take a deep sniff of **Versus Donna** and you are enveloped in a very sexy embrace.

Wear bright, fruity colours with it and splashy prints, adding tons of faux jewellery and stilettos. And wear all this with drop-dead chic – day or night, every day of the year.

Gio
by Giorgio Armani

Giorgio really got it right this time! Although there's absolutely nothing wrong with his signature scent **Armani**, with its sweet and heady outpouring of floral passion, it hardly mirrored the spirit of his clothes, which are anything but voluptuous and opulent.

Years later comes **Gio**. It is a perfect perfumed extension of Armani's fashion style – understated, straight-forward and pared-down to the point of minimalism. As Armani himself said, '**Gio** is not banal!' From its simple parchment box to its sloping-shouldered no-frills bottle, **Gio** is pure Armani.

It is a perfume of tremendous elegance, a composition of extreme artistry. The top note is composed of warm and golden orange and mandarin smells. To underline the theme there is a mass of orange blossom and sun-warmed summer flowers, most notably tuberose. If tuberose normally brings tears not so much of joy but of aversion to your eyes, used in **Gio** it's an exception. Coming from the very depths, under all the murmurs of vanilla and amber and faint scatterings of spice, its scent is amazingly subtle.

The soft sensuality of **Gio** and its sunny warmth make it a very Italian perfume, redolent of the countrysides of Sicily and Tuscany and the outgoing friendliness of Rome. Its informality and unsnobby elegance are truly Armani, giving simplicity an unequalled eloquence. The Italians, of course, took it immediately to their wide-open hearts. So should you. But a word of warning – it's extremely tenacious, so don't overdo it!

What to wear it with, where and when

Even if you can't afford a real Armani, so many clothes have been borrowed, plagiarised or influenced by his chic simplicity, you're sure to find the right sort of thing for a casual, unfussy look. Cool neutrals through to pastels and vibrant but not flashy colours suit **Gio**. It loves beautifully informal occasions – anything that isn't sloppy or gauche. It's quite passable on the young and not offensive on the old, but its real territory is the young to mature woman who loves life, loves simplicity, and shines, like **Gio**, all year round.

Giorgio Beverly Hills
by Giorgio Beverly Hills

Way back in 1981 I received a euphoric postcard from a friend visiting Los Angeles. The thing she was so excited about was a new perfume, **Giorgio**, which had just been unleashed on America.

When she hit our shores again I met her at the airport. There was no mistaking the entrance she made wearing her new American fragrance. (I didn't have the heart to tell her then that *it* was wearing *her*!) That was my introduction to the controversial **Giorgio**, a perfume with an incredibly polarising power. In New York it was banned from certain uppity restaurants, an action which turned out to be in its favour, publicity-wise! Even now the battle still rages on in sporadic outbursts. Be all that as it may, **Giorgio** seems to have secured a cachet of loyal devotees.

For those less enamoured of the perfume, the main objection seems to be its all-too-obvious tenacity and uncommon strength: it doesn't seem to fade at all. It does contain enormous concentrations of essences, all combined at top velocity, as well as hefty aledehydic 'modern' notes. But that was the way it was meant to be. Apparently Gale Hayman, one of the owners of the glitzy Giorgio boutique, was sick of the light, fresh fragrances in vogue during the seventies. She was determined to introduce a multi-floral of epic dimensions. She scoured the world's top perfume houses and after much searching she found it – a perfume like a thunderbolt.

With its headlong assault of narcissus backed up with gardenia, tuberose, jasmine and orange blossom, plus a splash of mandarin and some aldehydic rose-like notes, **Giorgio** certainly is high-powered. Its arrangement of flowers and fruits is further electrified by the addition of ylang ylang, patchouli, nutmeg, orris root, sandalwood and a liberal dash of vetyver. With its passionate gusto, **Giorgio** was born to be in the limelight. Whatever you personally think of it, it is a most prodigal perfume.

What to wear it with, where and when

Giorgio was born for the bright lights, so it dazzles with yellows, sharp greens and blues, brilliant white, flashy gold and electric colours. It's great for attracting attention at big occasions and is wonderful with extravagant dresses, though it's also quite comfortable with sporty and casual wear, designer jeans and the like. Great on blondes and redheads, as long as your dark roots don't show close up!

Havana pour elle
by Aramis

*I*n an unusual reversal of perfume procedure, Aramis introduced its men's fragrance in 1995, and later followed it up with a female companion, **Havana pour elle**. Both have a common deominator – strength! These are fragrances you don't overdo.

Havana pour elle is a sumptuous, ultra-heady affair. Persistent and powerful, it does not insinuate. Instead it takes you by the throat with a lush and sultry mix of flowers, fruits and spices, a lot of them extremely rare and never used in perfume before. There's night-blooming cereus, clementine, Caribbean raintree flower and the rare Queen of the Night orchid with its distinct vanilla character, plus marigold, daphne, heliotrope, lily of the valley and magnolia blossom garlanded around the lusciousness of mango, cabasa melon and pineapple. Then, in an almost impossible attempt to soften this volcanic eruption of exotica, come sandalwood, amber and vanilla bean. In all, it's a pretty explosive cocktail.

But despite this, **Havana pour elle** manages not to overpower you completely. With its smooth ebb and flow, its flirtatious and tantalising rhythms, it's reminiscent of what Havana must have smelt like when it was the capital of Caribbean swank, mystery, danger and sensuality. It's seductive, bold and assertive, which is why you shouldn't be too liberal with it. Its message and its staying power are anything but subtle.

What to wear it with, where and when

Think of Hollywood vamps like Lauren Bacall, Rita Hayworth, Hedy Lamarr and Lana Turner in their drop-dead glamourous heydays and you'll get the **Havana pour elle** message. Slink and sleek are the go, in over-the-top lamé, satin, taffeta, lace and anything transparent. Colours must be a tropical riot – nothing quiet or shy. Wear it afternoon to evening, and never in a cold climate. **Havana pour elle** loves splashy parties, seductive situations and anything by moonlight, as long as it's not too elegant. It's strictly for the mature woman, but only if she's a prowler.

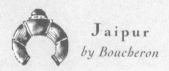

Jaipur
by Boucheron

*B*oucheron seems to be at great pains not to categorise its new perfume as an oriental. Given that it is not loaded with the usual bazaar delights of patchouli, jasmine, musk and spices that most oriental perfumes trumpet, perhaps it can escape the category in much the same way that Guerlain's **Samsara** does.

Jaipur is a happy inspiration and, for once, doesn't fall under the shadow of its famed predecessor. It is not only wonderfully unalike **Boucheron**, it is also a totally successful and utterly captivating essay in the art of harmonising fruit and flowers with a delicacy and subtlety few perfumes of the same ilk have managed.

I suppose I should start by saying that the bottle is a knockout, but coming from Boucheron, that goes without saying. Inspired by the Indian Nauratan bracelet, an amulet studded with precious stones and worn by rich brides of Jaipur, it contains a masterful accord of shimmering freshness and soft sensuality.

From its gentle top notes of just-ripe plum, peach and apricot with the sweetness of freesia, to its heart that beats romantically but quite fiercely with dark roses, **Jaipur** could almost be called rhapsodic. But this deliciousness is then deepened with notes of iris and acacia, with a haunting echo of peony placed deeper in the *mélange*. It is then anchored in velvety oakmoss and mysterious heliotrope with musk, amber and sandalwood.

There's a sense of surrender to this perfume, with its serenity and its gentle intensity. It has a splendour that is not remotely vulgar, but as charming as a magical spell. I advise you to fall under it.

What to wear it with, where and when

No, you don't have to swan around in an Indian sari, but clothes that are relaxed, swathed, draped and generally wafty are ideal – clothes of an afternoon or evening style, luxurious and languid. Go for silks or anything that swishes into a room with maximum impact. Keep colours to serene blues and greens, ruby reds and purples, with flashes of gold and silver. Even the oft-neglected orange gets a look-in, but go for the apricot and nectarine shades rather than the volcanic ones. Naturally, if you have good big jewels, wear them – if not, invest in some stand-out faux stuff. It's a case of always being the sophisticated lady with **Jaipur**. Anyone from twenty-something on will feel the ensnaring effects of this cool-headed, quiet vamp.

Jardins de Bagatelle
by Guerlain

PRONUNCIATION:
zjhar-DAN duh bag-uh-TELL
gair-LARN

*F*irstly I must point out that this perfume comes in *eaux* forms only, and not as an *extrait* or concentrate. More's the pity! But it is of such strength for an *eau* that Guerlain may have feared a full-strength version would be too explosive!

Jardins de Bagatelle is named after those beautiful gardens bordering the Bois de Boulogne in Paris – gardens that, since the days of the hapless Queen Marie Antoinette, have been planted with literally thousands upon thousands of roses, bulbs and flowering plants that practically cause an olfactory overload in spring and summer, such is the intensity of their combined scents.

This perfumed fugue of white flowers begins with a dominant solo flower note, that of the passionately perfumed trumpeting tuberose, which is then joined just as jubilantly by gardenia, rose, jasmine, magnolia and orange blossom. In the masterful hands of Guerlain, not one of these heady scents is allowed to out-shout the others. A harmonic unity is gracefully achieved, the effect of which is glorious.

More redolent of a warm summer's day than an innocent spring one, this perfume seems to excite, exhilarate and seduce by fanning out sinuously as if carried on a cooling breeze across freshly clipped green lawns. It seems to move with you like a second skin.

Being an *eau de parfum*, **Jardins de Bagatelle** never outstays its welcome, so you can envelop yourself lavishly in its sybaritic pleasures and feel you're wearing absolutely nothing but bliss!

What to wear it with, where and when

Jardins de Bagatelle is nothing like the Chelsea Flower Show, so don't go thinking that wearing anything flowery will do. This is no retiring English rose you're dealing with but an exquisite and passionate Gallic fantasy. It needs lovely and romantic clothes and colours, in fine fabrics, whether dressy or carefully casual. Perfect with white or cream, pastels, greens and blues, from ultra-pale to ultra-vivid, it's lovely to wear day and night and it positively blossoms at twilight. It's a perfume that's perfectly happy to go anywhere. Age is immaterial, so you can spray away or splash it around and be in your private Garden of Eden.

Jean-Paul Gaultier
by Jean-Paul Gaultier

PRONUNCIATION: zjhon-POLE GO-tee-ay

*N*ever judge a perfume by its packaging, especially this bombshell from the most eccentric *couturièr* in Paris! Thriving on his *enfant terrible* image, Gaultier took great pains to ensure that his signature perfume would shock the pants off the pundits and leave his league of adoring fans in ecstasy.

Apparently he chose half a dozen or so awesome 'noses' to sit around the conference table and nut out the ground rules he expected to be broken. He managed to flummox them all by wandering off into a nostalgic reverie about his grandmother and all the sweet smells that surrounded her and haunted him still.

He also droolingly drew on his memories and delight at discovering a pink satin girdle (with *décolleté* and suspenders) in her closet. From these rather disparate inspirations of the old world he sought to re-create his childhood in a perfume that would satisfy today's eclecticism. And eclectic is the word for the finished product.

It's presented in what is probably the most arresting packaging since Elsa Schiaparelli's **Shocking**. One is first confronted by what looks like an unlabelled can of salmon with *Jean-Paul Haute Parfumerie* stamped in no-frills cargo lettering over it. Lift off the lid and, lo and behold, there's gran's corset on a very voluptuous torso!

Now have a spray of the perfume. What would you expect? An explosion of volatile scents to knock your socks off? Wrong. **Jean-Paul Gaultier** smells exactly like you might remember your dear old granny's scent: sweet and powdery and innocent as a cherub's chubby cheeks. Roses and orange blossom and Florentine iris burst into your unprepared nostrils – heady and penetrating. Then comes lots of sensuous vanilla, old-world musk and a spice-charge of ginger and star anise. As the final coup there's a delicate pervasion of rare orchid.

If all this sounds cloying, it isn't. Somehow it amounts to a sweet synergism that smells disarmingly ladylike. It's not radical, but frankly sentimental!

What to wear it with, where and when

Despite its quirkiness, treat **Jean-Paul Gaultier** as you would any other perfume that may attract you. You don't have to wear anything outrageous. Stick to either bright, clear colours or romantic prints and pastels. It's a knockout at snappy dinner parties and the cocktail crush and is even lively enough to wear outdoors. Though a washout in winter, come spring and summer this curiously sweet perfume weaves a potent spell. Wearing **Jean-Paul Gaultier** comes down to this: if you're in the mood for it, then that's the right time. I promise you you won't feel grandmotherly!

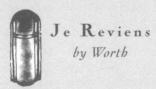

Je Reviens
by Worth

Two things the French have a great respect for are flowers and francs. The more of each, the better. The flower farmers in the sunny south and the villagers of a tiny hamlet called Lozere rely on both rare flowers and subsequent francs for their livelihood. Each year since 1932 they have gathered for the Parisian House of Worth two flowers vital to the continuing production of the unique and classic **Je Reviens** – the iris root and wild narcissus, which has a much more beautiful fragrance than its cultivated cousin. They're never likely to become rich from these fickle pickings, but as long as **Je Reviens** is made from these natural ingredients, they're ensured of a regular income.

Once in the hands of the perfumers, these two priceless glories are mixed with jasmine, orange blossom, vetyver and carnation, with a dash of ylang ylang and tuberose as well. Thus emerges the miraculous smell recognisable immediately as the great **Je Reviens** – 'I am returning'. Its effect is difficult to describe, since it seems to develop separately but simultaneously on two distinct levels. One level is mysterious and woody, with piquant flashes of herbs; the other is a heady rush of flowers in happy profusion. The mix gradually merges to become both disturbing and poignant, youthful and radiant. Because it's such a rarity in perfume, the French treasure **Je Reviens** as a superior example of their supreme superiority in these matters of taste, and it's no wonder they thumb their noses with typical Gallic contempt at foreign perfumers who try to emulate the sassy insouciance of such a classic.

There's no doubt that this is a perfume for the young, but its lightness and *joie de vivre* give lie to its monumental complexity and superb balance, which is why it possesses such a deeply emotional elusiveness. It's not to be treated like so much froth and bubble, nor is it wise to expect it to endow you with endearing young charms either. Sensible women who might be a touch past its magnetism are best advised to give it to daughters – never to your mother-in-law, though. She'll suspect you're trying to take the micky out of her!

What to wear it with, where and when

Since it's really only for the under thirties, the obvious colour choices are all blues, violets, lots of white and the lighter versions of yellow, green and pink. Prints, stripes, spots or anything happy and light-hearted are fine with it, and it can be worn with ease at any hour of the day or night, any season of the year. It's especially relaxed with casual clothes and loves to accompany pretty little dresses to parties. **Je Reviens** adores company and bright gatherings – it's not a pensive perfume. It's also wonderful in the bath, and loves to be layered.

Jicky
by Guerlain

*W*ould you believe that this perfume, which has practically become a household name in perfumed circles, was launched in 1889? *Vraiment!*

Aimé Guerlain rocked the perfume world and created history at the same time by being the first perfumer to have the audacity to use synthetic oils in perfume. While it shocked the pantaloons off society with its 'ferociously modern' smell, **Jicky** became not only a chemical breakthrough, it was also honoured as the first of *'Les Grands Parfums'*.

Even now a quick rundown of its components comes as something of a surprise. It's a truly innovative mix of lavender and bergamot with hesperides (citrus oils) and sandalwood, the punch of pungent basil and rosemary, and *bois de rose,* a rosewoody smell derived from a synthetic. I've also heard there's a hint of jasmine and Florentine iris in the perfume, plus a breath of *fougère* (French fern) in the middle background as well as civet, amber and vanilla for the anchor notes. This wouldn't surprise me, especially not the vanilla, which became Guerlain's subtle signature in nearly all the House's later perfumes.

Jicky has an unrivalled honesty. It also has the great power possessed by great perfumes – to be able to evoke nostalgic memories at a single whiff. A woman I know recently bought it for her mother, who thought it had long vanished from the scene. The eighty-year-old woman was astonished to be greeted by a wonderful flood of memories that brought smiles and tears to her face. She had worn **Jicky** as a mere teenager!

Aimé Guerlain too may have associated his perfume with a memory. Rumour has it that it was in remembrance of a love found and lost with a beautiful English girl that he created **Jicky**. There are no prizes for guessing what her nickname was!

What to wear it with, where and when

This perfume was made for the lover of the outdoors: after a hectic game on the court or a bracing cross-country ride, a splash of it will do wonders! Being a daylight sprite, **Jicky** adores sporty and casual clothes – nothing too dressy, unless you're young, in which case you can wear it with practically anything! Its favourite colours are white, cream, navy, all the sharp blues, greens and yellows, plus geranium, orange and ginger. Pastels aren't strong enough for its brash vivacity. Age and seasons don't matter to it much, and it's marvellous to have on hand when you feel quite jaded with perfumes of more serious intent.

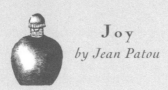

Joy
by Jean Patou

J have a friend who firmly believes in the adage 'if you have it, flaunt it'. Since she has ample to flaunt, she has little problem making it centre-stage and finding herself surrounded by admiring males who spend a lot of time darting sly glances down her considerable cleavage. But, like most women surrounded by admiring males, she's strictly a one-man woman, and like most one-man women she sticks with religious fervour to one perfume – the one she was wearing when he proposed! In her case it was **Joy**.

Some women seem destined to wear this perfume with such success. Others merely aspire to its haughty grandeur. Others again feel quite confronted by its outspokenness. So **Joy** is not every woman's joy! Nevertheless, when it was launched in 1931 the social set wore it like a uniform. An entire world of women succumbed to its charms and clamoured for their men to buy it for them. And men did, because they loved the smell of it as well.

When Jean Patou created his perfume he used a stunning concentration of Grasse jasmine and Bulgarian roses that simply out-perfumed any other similar alliances. Over this voluptuous bed he spread a hundred essences of other flowers (all a secret, still) and finished off the entire lethal cocktail with animal civet as a fixative. That's why **Joy** never seems to fade ungracefully away.

Over the course of the sixty-odd years of its life, **Joy** has not changed one iota. It has never lowered its sights, never altered its highly secret formula. To many it is synonymous with the glamorous world of opulent luxe. I, for one, agree. It is ageless, seasonless, and perfect at almost any occasion. It is tantalising, mesmerising, seductive and supremely confident. Above all, it is ravishingly beautiful.

What to wear it with, where and when
Go for the spectacular stuff of bright pink, heliotrope, scarlet, black, black and white, gold, and anything metallic. **Joy** is fabulous with evening wear, cut as low as it goes, and is a perfect counterpoint to snappy suits and dramatic dresses. Wonderful at big gatherings, **Joy** was born to party. It's also spectacular on not-so-innocent brides.

Kenzo
by Kenzo

Kenzo likens his beautiful signature perfume to the art of Ikebana – that intricately simple way of arranging flowers, fruits, woods, moss and pebbles into a perfectly balanced entity. Traditionally this is achieved in three stages: Shi-ki, sensuous images of white summer flowers; Otsoyou, a sense of delicious tranquillity from scented trees; and Issa, flower and fruit fragrances combining for a mysterious new synthesis.

One can compare the three traditional occidental stages of a perfume's unfolding on the wearer – the top, centre and base notes – to the oriental synthesis, thus making **Kenzo** the epitome of an artful arrangement of scents. Strictly speaking it is not an oriental type, but the influence is there in more ways than one. It is composed of a vast bouquet of strong-scented white flowers and richly delicious fruits with overlays of mosses, woods and spices.

The flowers, all pristine and pure, are intoxicating knockouts – tuberose, magnolia, gardenia, jasmine and ylang ylang. They're garlanded with plum and peach and laced with orange, mandarin and bergamot, then wreathed in oakmoss and iris and softly underlined with sandalwood, coriander and cardamom. Finally, a veil of musk and vanilla is drawn gently over the arrangement. If it sounds mesmerising, it certainly is – so intoxicating it becomes an intangible but sensual fantasy.

Kenzo is strong and clinging, its heady notes of tuberose and plum dominating as it settles on the skin. It is enshrined in a slightly oblique pebble-shaped bottle of frosted glass topped with an abstracted full-blown rose. The effect of bottle and perfume is one of unique symmetry – an exquisitely balanced arrangement.

What to wear it with, where and when

Kenzo is rich and elegant and is therefore the domain of the sophisticated woman. It loves well-cut but adventurous clothes that are set well apart from the usual. They may be day, afternoon or evening clothes, but never sporty or casual. **Kenzo** loves interesting new ways with fine wool, delicate cotton, linen, voile, silk – nothing heavy or opulent. The same applies to its favourite colours, which are vibrant but not flashy: orange, yellow, rose pink, violet, chocolate, ginger, cream and white. It's an occasion perfume, impressing with its quiet beauty and exquisite refinement. It blooms most vividly at night when the breezes stir the white flowers, giving off a disturbing and hypnotic intoxication. Don't underestimate its Japanese connotations – **Kenzo** is anything but ephemeral.

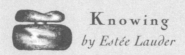

Knowing
by Estée Lauder

PRONUNCIATION: ESS-tay LOR-da

Knowing reminds me of those old-time wise-cracking New Yorkers – like Lauren Bacall in *How To Marry A Millionaire*, or Bette Davis in *All About Eve* – brittle, brilliant, bitchy. It has that same hard-shell exterior and pushover interior beloved of sleek, polished sophisticates. It's what Americans call 'high-toned', 'swanky' or 'classy' – formidable but basically friendly.

The inspiration for this perfume reputedly took place at Cap d'Antibes, where Mr and Mrs Evelyn Lauder were holidaying. Evelyn apparently wandered out onto the terrace to enjoy a balmy and fragrant Riviera breeze and smelt something wondrously mysterious – a warm, rich scent she couldn't identify. She and Mr Lauder followed their noses to a green bush full of tiny white flowers with an enchanting perfume. The next day they tracked its origins down, revealing it as pittosporum.

Back in New York, Evelyn pressed ahead with the making of a new Lauder scent. To pittosporum's rich powers she added some other typical Provençale flowers, like tuberose, rose, jasmine, lily of the valley, orange flower, marigold and the much underrated mimosa. For a touch of the Orient, ylang ylang was called upon, along with a battalion of oakmoss, vetyver, amber, patchouli, musk, clove, bayleaf and, finally, rich vanilla. But something more was needed for a warmer and sunnier embrace synonymous with the south of France, and it turned out to be the ripeness of melon and plum. Personally I think it's their delicious inclusion that gives **Knowing** its sensuous magnetism, its upbeat modernity and intelligent charm.

But attractive and poised as it may be, **Knowing** belongs to the woman who is a breed apart. She is not averse to glamour, as long as it's not cheap. She has a certain appreciation of her subtly wielded power, but never flaunts it. Her intrinsic intuition guides her in the other direction where she can charm the angels and get away with it by laughing at herself. She is wise, witty and wonderful. As they say on Broadway, 'She's quite a dame!'

What to wear it with, where and when

Clothes should be sleek, slick and underplayed. **Knowing** hates tizziness and unnecessary glitter; its glamour is more refined. Silk jersey, chiffon, satin, taffeta, velvet, organza and suede are all fine, in muted colours like vanilla, tobacco, peach, moss green, hazy blue and ruby red. Keep accessories down to a bare-but-beautiful minimum and be excessively well groomed and polished. **Knowing** is lovely to wear at home but loves select gatherings as well, as long as the guest list is witty and clever. It's versatile enough to weather all seasons but is to be avoided by the young.

L'Air du Temps
by Nina Ricci

**PRONUNCIATION: lair du TOM
NEEN-a REECH-ee**

Every time I smell this enchanting perfume I think of the paintings of Botticelli — nymph-like ladies with garlanded tresses, diaphanous dresses billowing in the breeze, their graceful curves enticingly placed against rippling leaves and water. **L'Air du Temps** gives exactly that impression.

Everything about this perfume is rapturous, from its famous Lalique doves serving as a stopper for the sinuously curved and fluted bottle, to the enchanted gathering of flowers and spices that give **L'Air du Temps** its unique angelic aura. Since its introduction in 1945, women have fallen completely under its gentle spell. And so they should.

No other perfume has achieved its delicate balance of strongly scented flowers with a gentle overlay of spices that breathe a tantalising murmur of the exotic into what is basically a beautiful bouquet of rose, carnation, jasmine, gardenia, violet and ylang ylang. Wraiths of sandalwood, vetyver and ambergis give **L'Air du Temps** its gentle persistence. It has a lilting, elusive presence that never sours or stales but simply and modestly fades away sweetly on the air. The spice ingredients are handled with such discreet artistry and so subtly blended it's nigh on impossible to isolate any one, let alone identify the entire litany. And in this case I think the mystery is better than unromantic dissection.

L'Air du Temps is the sort of perfume that ingratiates itself on the wearer with its delicacy, fragility and sheer fascination. It evokes the memories of summer afternoons alive with the promise of romance and adventure, or tender twilights when we all wish the sun would never set. That's the enticing poignancy of L'Air du Temps – its magical ability to make you feel young, vulnerable and submissive – like Botticelli's Venus emerging from the rippled waters on her scalloped shell.

What to wear it with, where and when

It's pastels and purples only for L'Air du Temps, the latter in every shade from palest lavender to heliotrope. Fabrics should be near-transparent, or crisp and clean. It's wonderful day or night, and can cope sweetly with almost any occasion. This is a perfume of innocent mystery, so let it speak sweetly for itself – and you. While not strong enough for winter, it revels in the high spirits of spring and the languid loveliness of summer. Socially speaking, it adores parties and is at its pristine best at weddings. There won't be a dry eye in the church!

Laura
by Laura Biagiotti

PRONUNCIATION: LOW (as in wow!) -ra
bee-uh-gee-OTT-e

'*L*aura, it's your face in the misty light . . .' so the classic old standard goes. And the same might be said for this new perfume from one of Italy's best-loved *couturièrs*.

Laura is very misty indeed, and totally unlike its lustier sister perfumes, **Roma** and **Venezia**. It was inspired by the lovely lakes of northern Italy, thus much use is made of limpid blue waters and crystalline clarity in both the ambience and presentation of this ultra-feminine charmer. It's not the strident perfume you might expect from Biagiotti but a genteel fragrance of the fruity-flowery category.

The most unexpected thing about **Laura** is that it doesn't smell remotely Italian: there is nothing flamboyant, dazzling or outrageous about it. If anything it veers toward the delicacy of some modern French concoctions. **Laura**'s message is one of inner calm and serenity. An initial whiff of fresh watermelon, white peach and lychee confirms this. The heart is underlaid quietly with flowers, predominantly freesia and waterlily, with hints of violet, rose petals, Florentine iris and camellia. Again the effect is delicate rather than effusive, with the freesia standing out just a little to make a harmonic accent with the watermelon. The base is also very subtle, with soft notes of juniper, fern, sandalwood, vetyver and the merest dash of vanilla. It's actually this base with its sense of faraway places that gives **Laura** its depth and long-lastingness.

It is a most becoming but subtle perfume, fascinating enough to radiate that face in the misty light with a sense of tranquillity. In that respect, it is quite reminiscent of the Italian lakes at their most peaceful – which, these days, is usually only in the dead of night!

What to wear it with, where and when

Laura is emphatically a spring and summer perfume, so its colours lean to the light and bright – blues, greens, yellows, pinks, creams and white – as pale or as vibrant as you like. Clothes in cotton, silk, chiffon, georgette and linen are the go, with emphasis on the diaphanous and floaty. It's fine with classy casuals as much as dreamy concoctions for afternoon and evening wear – and a knockout with lacy lingerie. Because it's such an intensely feminine perfume it does well in intimate situations, being too discreet to shout its praises at more hectic gatherings. It smells as delicious on a teenager as it does on a dowager far from the madding crowd. It will not sit easily on the woman who is totally extroverted or flashy. I hardly think she'd be attracted to the beguiling subtlety of **Laura** anyway.

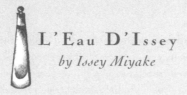

L'Eau D'Issey
by Issey Miyake

A Japanese designer conquering Paris *couture* with his fearless innovation and minimalist concepts is extraordinary enough, but having the temerity to brief a perfumer on a fragrance idea that seemed not only absurd but impossible was really rising somewhat above one's station, even in the often bizarre creative Parisian melting pot. But then again, the designer in question was Issey.

In his inscrutable Japanese way, Issey Miyake is nothing if not insistent and imaginative, not troubling himself over limitations that get in the way of his vision. Nevertheless, a lot of eyes were raised heavenwards when he announced he wanted his very first perfume – his signature scent – to smell like water! How could a perfume smell like scentless water? But Issey insisted, and at last his vision was realised.

Of course, **L'Eau D'Issey** doesn't smell like water – more like a perfume with the *purity* of fresh water. This is achieved by using pure white flowers: freesias, cyclamens, lilies, tuberose stems and (so it goes!) camellias. The sea also comes to the rescue with ozonic notes that are miles away from the outspoken ones used in Dior's **Dune** but which are nonetheless redolent of sun, sand and surf. Then there's the unblemished purity of edibles – a blush of peach or apricot and a surprisingly bold whiff of sliced cucumber.

Distilled to a highly refined liquid, this perfume stands out like a sentinel symbolising the purity of life itself, albeit with a rather pronounced edge of worldly sensuality. And L'Eau D'Issey manages to *look* like a sentinel as well, with its cone-shaped bottle topped by a globular water droplet perched like a beacon atop a lighthouse! Stunning, and already considered a collector's item.

L'Eau D'Issey is a lovely fragrance, though slightly over-tenacious, so do be sparing. It may have captured the essence of purity itself, but in reality it's pure dynamite!

What to wear it with, where and when

L'eau D'Issey loves lots of pure bright white, shimmering silver, pale pale grey, transparent amethyst, soft apricot and peach, sea green and ice blue in any fabric that's delicately translucent and diaphanous. It loves frail watercolour prints, vague florals and quivering stripes, especially softly metallic ones. Don't bother it with anything tailored or remotely spectacular – it much prefers the freedom of strikingly individual clothes. L'Eau D'Issey works its spell best in very intimate situations. The young were born for it, the more mature can succumb and adapt to its simplistic nature, but it may induce floods of nostalgic tears on the elderly. Keep it for spring and summer and lock it away in the cooler months. And don't just display it – *wear* it!

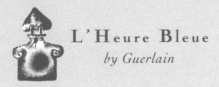

L'Heure Bleue
by Guerlain

PRONUNCIATION: ler BLER
gair-LARN

*V*ery, very few perfumes have survived two world wars and countless changes of tastes and fashions, but **L'Heure Bleue**, created in 1912, has managed it. Though it has almost given up the ghost as far as recapturing its once mass popularity is concerned, it still has a very devoted following by women of discerning taste.

When Jacques Guerlain composed this complex, magnificent perfume in 1912, it epitomised the languid world of the privileged. It is said that because he had premonitions of the awful war to come, he imbued **L'Heure Bleue** with a nostalgic tranquillity – his heartfelt tribute to a beloved way of life about to vanish forever.

L'Heure Bleue is a little like an Impressionist painting of Paris by twilight, its edges blurred with the soft evocation of light and shade and shimmering, smoky reflections. It is a perfume of repose named for that magical blue hour that hovers over the city with a palpable, vibrating hush, the sun just out of sight and the sky trailed with apricot and rose.

In composition it starts with an extraordinary balance of lush Bulgarian roses over soft citrus notes of bergamot.

Then the distant throbbing murmur of jasmine, orris root and heliotrope infiltrate over the lovely Herbe de la Saint Jean, with the sweet sensuousness of musk and the familiar Guerlain trademark of vanilla coming last to give the perfume the slightest *frisson* of oriental exotica. This fabulous masterpiece of blending is one of Guerlain's crowning achievements – a mesmerising, harmonic entity.

It's not an easy perfume to wear. Far from being merely lyrical or romantic, it is infinitely wistful, totally individualistic and irresistibly mesmerising. I fervently hope its devotees will not only keep wearing it, but inititate others into its mysteries and beauties so it will never, never disappear into the blue void of unavailability.

What to wear it with, where and when

No prizes for guessing that blue in nearly all its glorious guises is the ideal companion for **L'Heure Bleue**. Perhaps navy might be dismissed, but the misty, cloudy, shadowy, smoky, faraway blues (especially in clothes of filmy femininity) are perfect for its mysteries. All the shrouded, shadowy colours like dusky rose, muted grey, sage, pearl, lilac and *crème café* are suitable too. As far as personality goes, the woman who'll fall under the spell of **L'Heure Bleue** will be a dreamer, a softly-spoken seducer, a lover of subtlety. She could be young or old or in-between – it makes no difference as long as she possesses true elegance.

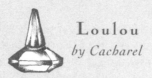

Loulou
by Cacharel

*A*naïs Anaïs is a pretty hard act to follow, but Jean Cacharel made a wise decision in moving to the opposite end of the emotional spectrum with his second perfume. **Loulou** is as worldly-wise as **Anaïs Anaïs** is all innocence.

Perfumer Jean Guichard imbued in **Loulou** the essence of the hedonistic, sin-for-sin's sake early twenties. His, or Cacharel's, inspiration was the classic silent film *Pandora's Box*, starring the enigmatically beautiful American actress Louise Brooks. Her performance as the fated Lulu is the epitome of the manslayer, the temptress, the girl-woman who lives for the thrill of the moment. Which is why **Loulou** has been tagged a *jeune femme fatale* perfume.

It's actually a very complex and compelling oriental. Decorated with smouldering flowers, it uses the rare and elusive tiare blossom as its ephemeral pivot. Growing in the tropical Pacific Islands, the tiare is a small gardenia-like flower with a sweetly heady perfume. In **Loulou** its haunting essence is overlaid with cherry-like heliotrope and the seductiveness of ylang ylang, orange flower, jasmine and iris. Then the really big guns are brought out to fire a wild salvo of vanilla, sandalwood, incense, cassia, bergamot and the sultry, caramel-scented tonka bean – a real Pandora's Box if ever there was one!

Loulou, in its intense lapis lazuli blue pyramid-shaped bottle, trumpets out its message loud and clear, becoming more and more passionate and provocative until reaching its torrid, inevitable climax. If all this is too much for you, try the new **Loulou Blue**. It's a little less strident than its sister, but still pretty powerful.

What to wear it with, where and when

Since it's a perfume primarily for the young, **Loulou** needs streetsmart, rather feckless clothes. On the other hand, it's too grown-up and worldly for jeans and T-shirts, so give **Loulou** its due with simple, drop-dead gear. Being a perfume for the evening it likes black and dark blue, with electric shocks of teal, scarlet, copper, orange, silver white, steel grey and shiny green. It loves leather, net, lace, velvet and slinky satin, so forget the filmy approach. **Loulou** means business – seductive business – and since sensuousness isn't seasonal, neither is it. To wear **Loulou** properly you must have a coquettish air of being up to no good. Really, though, beneath the mask, you're all childish innocence.

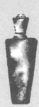

Madame Rochas
by Rochas

PRONUNCIATION: mud-ARM hro-SHAR

Such was the popularity of Marcel Rochas's striking *haute couture* in the late forties that at one never-to-be-forgotten party in Paris the entire gathering of socialites went into a brouhaha when no fewer than eight women made their separate entrances wearing the same Rochas dress! Rest assured, however, that even if you are one of eight women in the same place wearing this Rochas perfume, all hell will probably *not* break loose. **Madame Rochas** is not the kind of perfume that stops people dead in their tracks. It's far too well bred for that.

Launched in 1960 by the widow of Rochas, the elegant Hélène, **Madame Rochas** very quickly became the flagship perfume of the House. It was also declared a 'classic' by perfume noses and established a fond place in French hearts with its softly aspirational emotions and romantic elegance.

To maintain its air of being at one with modern lifestyles it has recently undergone a little corrective surgery to add even more sparkle and wit. Some soft new aldehydes have been called in, revitalising and bringing into sharp focus the rich floral tapestry of the original. The overall smell is still conceived of Bulgarian roses and jasmine with tuberose, narcissus and ylang ylang. There's also some wildly sweet honeysuckle, as well as a touch of violet-like orris and orange blossom for further sunny lightness. But **Madame Rochas** still maintains her secret magnetism with cedar and musk throwing their veils of fascination over the other ingredients.

All of this Parisian poise and femininity is brought to a climax typical of the Rochas style: it is presented with lovely simplicity in an octagonal cylindrical bottle, a reproduction of an eighteenth century crystal *flacon* tastefully decorated with motifs from an antique French tapestry. All very refined indeed! But, never fear, with **Madame Rochas**'s recent petite operation, she's a new woman with modern attitudes and a younger outlook on life – so she's more than ready to kick up her high heels!

What to wear it with, where and when

Madame Rochas is not aloof but likes plenty of action, sophisticated wit and laughter. Clothes should be smart but daring, with patterns, prints, large old-rose florals and tapestries in satin, taffeta and silk. Colours such as wine red, caramel, oyster, toffee, moss green, cyclamen and black are perfect. Even neutrals pass muster. The young automatically avoid **Madame Rochas**, but smart mature women with dignity and a twinkle in the eye are naturals for it. Autumn and winter are its best times, and it deserves only the most civilised and feminine occasions.

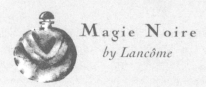

Magie Noire
by Lancôme

PRONUNCIATION: mar-zjhee NWAH
LARN-com

Black magic this perfume most certainly is! Recently I was at a dinner party when a guest arrived a little late. Two other people in the room were French. The minute the elegantly dressed guest walked in, they both said ecstatically, 'Ah! **Magie Noire**!' That's how unmistakable and admired a fragrance it is – on the right woman.

Magie Noire has a compelling, provocative presence. It requires a woman with style, poise and a certain mystery to fully reveal its dynamics. Its formulation is a most unusual one. Instead of starting with an extravagant floral bouquet like most perfumes, it opts for a strong woody approach backed by amber-laced flowers. These woods – cedar and sandal – give it an earthy warmth sparked with quite a dazzling array of herbs and spices. Over all this comes the rich and refined seduction of beautiful Bulgarian roses in full bloom and a piquant splash of green Persian galbanum, which draws you deeper into the forest where the witchcraft is completed with a touch of potent patchouli and musk.

To call it sensual is an understatement. It quite clearly evokes a smouldering but fascinating witchery, but one which is more bewitching than dangerous. I don't think people will fall at your feet to do your bidding, but you can bet they'll be highly intrigued by this worldly, civilised but tantalising perfume.

What to wear it with, where and when

Black, what else? You could also wear it with dark grey, indigo, navy, purple, deep crimson, dark green and silver. I wouldn't advise wearing **Magie Noire** for afternoon teas, Christenings or weddings, but it might add a touch of sorcery to funerals. If you're the seductive type, by all means wear it for a job interview, but not after you've got the job: you won't be trusted by your colleagues! **Magie Noire** is definitely only for fully fledged temptresses, not young hopefuls.

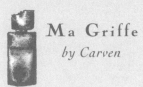

Ma Griffe
by Carven

PRONUNCIATION: mar-GREEF

kar-VAN

*I*t always amazes and saddens me when a perfume, especially one which has been so successful in the past it's become a part of perfume parlance, falls out of fashion. Whatever the reason for such a decline, it's a crying shame to see a perfume of **Ma Griffe**'s pedigree fade away to olfactory oblivion. Thank heavens, though, it hasn't quite come to that yet, and I hope a reacquaintance with its many charms will rekindle its flickering flame.

Ma Griffe has been a favourite with thousands of women for more than fifty years now. Launched in 1946, it was an immediate postwar success with its smart green-and-white striped packaging, its bold and clean-lined bottle, its air of vivacious and light-hearted elegance and, most of all, its utterly new style of composition.

Although basically a chypre-type perfume of the green family, with a hefty swag of flowers behind the bushes, **Ma Griffe** broke with tradition by using sharp green wood notes obtained from dazzling new synthetics. This gave it a thoroughly modern air akin to the hugely successful **Miss Dior** which was to appear hot on its heels.

At first encounter the top notes of **Ma Griffe** ('My Signature') are quite shattering and volatile. There's a sudden rush of gardenia, green leaves, citrus and clary sage (a herb with a peculiar mint-lavender smell) which becomes even more tumultuous in the middle section with lots of rose, jasmine, ylang ylang, neroli, vetyver and orris. Then come the softer base notes of oakmoss, sandalwood, cinnamon, amber and musk to anchor the entire avalanche in a dazzling exuberance. It's all quite breathtaking!

I think of **Ma Griffe** as a very 'smart' perfume – one that gives sharper definition to a woman of distinctive and witty personality. It is racy, snappy, happy and giddy, but far from frivolous or shallow. It positively exudes Parisian chic and panache but with tons of good-natured taste, not superficial posing. And that's not a bad signature to have!

What to wear it with, where and when

Ma Griffe comes pretty close to being a perfume for all women in all seasons. It's as fetching on the young as it is on the mature and it takes no notice of weather or time, its versatility fitting it out favourably for most occasions. **Ma Griffe**'s boundless optimism and joy should be enhanced by clear, bright colours, especially green, yellow, red, orange and white. It's also sensational with black and navy blue. Clothes should be simple, clean-lined, direct and smartly sophisticated. Anything safe is simply a waste of time with it. I think **Ma Griffe** is best on blondes and redheads, but don't let that stop you.

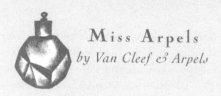

Miss Arpels
by Van Cleef & Arpels

PRONUNCIATION: ar-PELL

I cannot imagine a young woman who possesses poise and panache failing to go bananas over this wonderfully youthful and effervescent perfume. Sure, it has all the luxe that goes with its pedigreed name, but it has something else that I think is even more desirable – unbridled vivacity!

Miss Arpels is one of those rare new perfumes that reaches out and invites you into its charmed circle. It is utterly irresistible without being the slightest bit demanding. It merely flutters its lashes at you, winks and smiles and, if you're the right girl, you're done for! **Miss Arpels** is not a perfume you're intrigued or fascinated by. It's one you simply fall in love with, and stay in love with. What more could a girl ask for?

Its top notes are a big surprise. They rush straight to your head, and while you're trying to decipher just what you've been hit with (would you believe basil, lemon and watermelon?), the big floral guns are wheeled in to fire a scented barrage of jasmine and freesia backed by the delicious muskiness of sweet angelica. This takes the sharp edge off the first impression but doesn't by any means dull its zing. But this is not the whole bag of tricks of clever **Miss Arpels**. Underscoring the fruit and flower *mélange* come four beautiful soft notes to give body and soul to the perfume – velvety oakmoss, creamy sandalwood, luscious peach and sweet vanilla. It all sounds like the ingredients for some ambrosial dessert, which is just about right.

Miss Arpels is not the serious type, but nor is she capricious or frivolous. Underneath all her youthful facade, she's more than enticing – she's downright provocative. So watch out!

What to wear it with, where and when

'Miss' (or 'Young Ms', if you must) is the operative word. If you're over thirty, forget trying to force the youthful charms of **Miss Arpels** on your maturity; go for its older sisters (**First** or **Van Cleef**) instead. This is a perfume that revels in sassy, vivacious clothes in sassy, vivacious colours. It loves unstructured dresses, suits, sarongs, swirly skirts and dramatically low tops – anything provocative without being obviously seductive. Colours should be on the light but bright side, in particular pastels, pink and white. Because of its youth, **Miss Arpels** is impervious to weather extremes, and therefore makes a great travelling companion. Like any smart young woman, this perfume ingratiates itself with loads of charm and dash.

Miss Dior
by Christian Dior

*R*emember the New Look? Apparently, if you were around the traps after 1947, you could hardly have avoided it. It was Christian Dior's celebration of the end of shortages, rationing and those ugly clothes that were *de rigueur* under wartime conditions. It liberated women, and it also etablished Dior as the shining new star of Paris *haute couture*. Suddenly skirts were real skirts, incredibly full and long, necklines plunged, jewellery dazzled in cascades of glitter, and the air was full of the sweet smell of Dior's very first perfume, **Miss Dior**.

Miss Dior has practically become a household word since those wonderful days of liberation, but not once has it betrayed its considerable age. It is as fresh, different, unexpected and innovative today as it was at its debut. It's rare indeed to find a woman, or a man, for that matter, who doesn't like it. Yet it's no fence-sitter. Quite the opposite!

Its composition is sumptuous – a lush arrangement of gardenia, jasmine, *rose de France* and narcissus gilded with assertive notes of bergamot and patchouli and elevated with chypre harmonies of galbanum, oakmoss and amber. It's the green note and the unusual soft aldehydes that steer it clear of the usual floral harmonies into wilder arpeggios. **Miss Dior** is a perfume that sings soaringly sweet and pure.

With this unique perfume Dior opened the way ahead to a new breed of lighter, more spontaneous perfumes that perfectly complemented the new age. As he wrote in his autobiography, 'Europe was tired of letting off bombs. All it wanted now was to let off fireworks!' That's precisely what **Miss Dior** did – and, thank God, still does!

What to wear it with, where and when

All the pastels, virginal white and the bright clear jewel colours in subtly shimmering organza, silk, georgette, chiffon, piqué, linen, lace and tulle are the preserve of **Miss Dior**. It's a waste of time with black, red, purple and sombre colours, and deadly with neutrals. It's also ill at ease with glitz and glamour, preferring beautifully cut evening gowns, smart cocktail dresses, snappy suits and expensive casuals – anything chic and not overbearing. It loves company, so all occasions seem to suit its charms, and it works wonders day or night in any season. It has that intrinsic Dior well-mannered delicacy and poise.

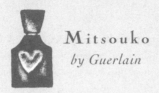

Mitsouko
by Guerlain

*M*itsouko is Japanese for 'mystery', and Guerlain's magical masterpiece, created in 1919, is just this – a hauntingly beautiful enigma.

With the cessation of the World War I there was a move toward lightness and tenderness. People craved simplicity and serenity. This coincided with the rediscovery of all things oriental, especially Japanese. Guerlain was responsive to all this when he made **Mitsouko**, but he also had another curious source of inspiration – the romance between a British naval officer and the wife of a Japanese admiral. The romance caused a scandal, and became the basis of a French best-seller, *La Bataille*. It was this love story and the mysteriously named woman, Mitsouko, that became the catalyst for Guerlain's fabulous new perfume.

After all these years, **Mitsouko** still shines in the Guerlain galaxy. Its main chord is emphatically green, with both eastern and western mosses in tandem with Sumatran vetyver and Sicilian bergamot. This greenness gives an overall impression of crushed forest leaves and dewy ferns. Underneath all this is a softly beautiful interlacing of peach and pear, jasmine and patchouli fanned with a warm amber finish and an infusion of elegant lilac blossom. This gloriously original composition assuages the senses with a totally hypnotic spell.

But **Mitsouko** is far from shy. In fact, it is quite assertive, sending out its subtle message at unexpected intervals, leaving behind a tranquil impression like delicate glass chimes tinkling in the wind.

On the right woman, **Mitsouko** is truly entrancing. As an ancient Japanese poet once wrote, 'one breath of her perfume and your city is lost. Another, and you forfeit a kingdom.'

What to wear it with, where and when

Mitsouko is enchanting with all greens, especially in silk, chiffon, organza, Chantilly lace and crêpe de Chine, and is equally lovely with sky blue, white and pale earthy colours. With black it's devastating! Age doesn't matter at all with it – even the relatively young can wear it well, and the very mature feel comfortable in its soft green envelopment. Like all beautiful things, **Mitsouko** has the enviable ability to sit gracefully and naturally through any occasion at any time, but it's at its most melting on langorous summer after-noons and romantic moonlit evenings. Aren't we all?

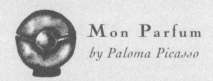

Mon Parfum
by Paloma Picasso

PRONUNCIATION: mon par-FUOM

pal-O-muh pik-AR-so

*P*aloma Picasso, the daughter of the great Spanish painter, has the distinctive, intense and almost arrogant carriage of her countrywomen overlaid with a dazzling armoury of striking features, including the famous red-slashed lips. The perfume she created is no less starkly sophisticated. In fact, it's a bombshell.

Paloma Picasso's instruction to her perfumer was to create 'something I would like to wear – warm, sophisticated, flamboyant, made to awaken the senses'. Whoever the genius was came up with the goods, bells ringing and flags flying. **Mon Parfum** is a knockout, completely unique and extraordinarily non-conformist. It uses chypre as a solid anchor on which to intertwine a mesmerising bouquet of strongly perfumed flowers – *rose de mai*, jasmine, deep-scented Bulgarian rose, earthy iris and romantic hyacinth. This is harmonised with a potent phalanx of such dynamos as ylang ylang, patchouli, sandalwood, oakmoss, amber and, best of all, a miraculous medley of mimosa, angelica and citrus oils, all fixed in the animal scent of civet! I suspect there's even a goodly thwack of tobacco leaf in there too.

Mon Parfum possesses that all-too-rare quality in new perfumes – audacity with good taste! It may have been created in France with an eye to the gigantic American market, but its ambience is distinctly Spanish – sunny, dramatic, passionate, imperious. It has something of the fiery flamenco about it – a tantalising sexual explicitness. It is strong (very) but with a hint of sweetness amid all its fireworks, making it easily approachable. If the gloriously rumbustious Ava Gardner were still with us, she'd no doubt be drawn to its intense evocation of clicking castanets, black lace mantillas, throbbing guitars and thunderous flamenco heels. *Olé!*

What to wear it with, where and when

Colours like scarlet, crimson, vermilion, black and gold are its natural companions, but so is white, vivid green, emerald, acid yellow, orange, hot pink, lime and indigo. Wear flashy dresses, tight pants, see-through blouses, leather, suede, satin, silk, taffeta, lace and plenty of jewellery. Be daring! Wear it day or night, winter and summer. It loves spectator sports, art galleries, ritzy restaurants, extravagant dinners and plush parties, and hates being left on its own anywhere. It's completely extroverted, and so must you be. If you're under twenty, wait a few years. Otherwise you can keep blasting away with it until they put you in a retirement village!

Moschino
by Moschino

PRONUNCIATION: moz-KEEN-o

*W*hat a sneaky little minx this one is! In its bottle it's all blushing pink and gilt innocence. With a red, white and blue ribbon around its neck, it looks for all the world like something you'd give your daughter at her debut.

Well, don't! Once released from its pristine packaging **Moschino** is a dervish! Like Salome and her infamous dance, it flashes waves of outright seduction. And it's no quick little striptease either: the performance goes on and on with the insistence of Ravel's *Bolero*.

Nothing prepared me for its onslaught the first time I smelt it. The bit of publicity I'd read must have been written by someone who'd got it mixed up with some other perfume. Words like 'gay', 'charming', 'flirtatious' and 'innocent' couldn't have been more off the mark!

Actually, **Moschino** has something of a split personality. It starts out with high-pitched, zingy top notes of coriander and oregano with green galbanum and French marigold. Once these settle in, it changes alarmingly, becoming a full-on vamp from the Orient with flashes of ripe plum, carnation, ylang ylang, gardenia, rose, jasmine, nutmeg and a dash of hot pepper. It all adds up to some pretty torrid choreography that's further heightened with musk and patchouli. But **Moschino** hasn't finished its dance yet! The last veil is saturated in that sexpot standby, vanilla, and so the dance whirls on to its inevitable climax.

Moschino has always aimed at upsetting traditions with his *couture*, and this very sexy young perfume goes right along with that feeling. After all, despite Rita Hayworth's attempts to convince us otherwise with her ladylike performance, Salome was simply a rebellious brat who could toss off a few fancy dance steps. What's more, she simply hated being overdressed!

What to wear it with, where and when

Moschino needs the Moschino look – chopped-off pants and shirts, skimpy boleros, and transparent midriffs in a mish-mash of fabrics, prints, colours and textures. Like its maker, this perfume invents its own shorthand fashion chic. Wear it with shiny black, blood red, gold, white and fluorescent colours. It needs a personality with no hang-ups, no pretensions; it certainly doesn't need anyone over twenty-five! Seasons aren't important to **Moschino**, since it's basically a non-daylight perfume. It loathes fresh air and anything in it!

Must de Cartier
by Cartier

PRONUNCIATION: MOOST
(or, in plain old English, 'MUST')
KART-ee-air

*T*he legendary House of Cartier stands implacably by its motto, 'The Art of Being Unique'. It was inevitable that among all the clever, imaginative and wildly expensive jewellery Cartier creates for the super-rich, a perfume for the not-so-rich would emerge with great success. And indeed it did. **Must de Cartier** made its suitably Gallic grand entrance at the Château de Versailles in 1981 and was immediately embraced by women – with or without a Cartier account.

Must looks as glamorous and precious as a jewel in its red, gold and amber packaging. Its presentation is so tasteful as to be almost daunting, but once you smell the perfume you discover that it is not showy, not dynamic, not confronting – just truly sensational. **Must** is blended with such consummate artistry it resolutely refuses to be categorised. To call it a soft floral oriental is to misunderstand its rich complexity, yet it is certainly based on an orientalistic idea of exotic florals – rose, carnation, jasmine, jonquil and orange blossom. Its wooded notes of sandalwood, vetyver and amber are there as an eastern influence, as are the Persian notes of rare citrus oils and vanilla. There's also a sharp note of lime leaves which leads into animal notes of civet, musk and ambergris.

Despite all this oriental sorcery, it's as if a jewelled veil were drawn over its ingredients to conceal its emotional depths from surface glitter and extravagance. This gives **Must** an enigmatic, elusive, unfathomable mysteriousness – a disturbing beauty you can play up to the hilt. Like all rare jewels, **Must** will glitter or smoulder to your whim.

What to wear it with, where and when

Real riches need neither embellishment nor advertising, so don't overdo it with clothes and colours. With **Must**, good taste is the golden rule. Don't ever insult it with casual or sporty clothes, and never wear it in broad daylight; wait at least until dusk. Keep it away from the youngsters. You may have to hide it from your mother, too, who could wear it quite elegantly. Seasons are of little importance, since riches rise to any occasion.

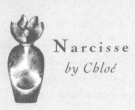

Narcisse
by Chloé

PRONUNCIATION: nar-SEASE

KLO-e

pparently when **Narcisse** was about to be launched, a dilemma arose over the question of its name. Had the perfume been named for the narcissus flower itself, or for the mythical Greek beauty who fell in love with his own reflection? In short, was it merely seductive, or was it a seducer?

To edge around a firm answer, let me begin by saying that **Narcisse** is decidely not a true narcissus perfume. It certainly has a fair whack of the floral fragrance in its formulation, but it is not the dominant note by a long way. That accolade goes to the rarely used plumeria, which is sometimes known as West Indian red jasmine but more correctly as the red frangipani. This gorgeous tropical beauty has a very sweet powdery perfume which is almost soporific in large doses. Mixed with rose and apricot, plus the pristine narcissus, its bouquet packs quite a punch, especially when bolstered with sandalwood, musk and the hypnotic vanilla bean. In total, **Narcisse**'s ingredients have a powerhouse effect, making the perfume both enticing and seductive and quite capable of mowing down any opposition with all guns blazing. Subtlety is not in its strong point, but it's certainly not vulgar, having an outgoing impact that's difficult to ignore. It's very tenacious, so don't swamp yourself in it. A little says all you need to say.

What to wear it with, where and when

Narcisse is a natural for romantic floral prints and bright colours, and can be quite charming with floaty dresses and dreamy lingerie. It can be worn day or night, at almost any occasion except a very grand one. Seasons don't worry it either, although it's best in spring and summer. **Narcisse** can stand up to plenty of passion and foreplay but is also quite content to be featured at home, as long as you're the bright and bubbly type. The young can get away with it but it is the mature who will find it a sweet, uncomplicated pleasure. I like it best on blondes – brunettes and redheads seem a bit glum in it.

No. 5
by Chanel

*N*o. 5 by Chanel (*not* 'Chanel No. 5') is the name most synonymous with the perception of perfume in people's minds. Despite the fact that it was created as long ago as 1921, **No. 5** has maintained its position at the top year after year.

Its genesis is less well known than its scent. It was in the early decades of this century, when Gabrielle Chanel was riding the crest of the *haute couture* wave with her revolutionary clothes, that she decided the House of Chanel should have its signature perfume, an idea almost unheard of at the time. She asked France's most innovative perfumer, Ernest Beaux, to create a perfume that would once and for all liberate women from prewar single-flower scents ('A woman should smell like a woman, not a rose!' she sniffed). Ernest Beaux presented Chanel with two groups of original ideas – the first numbered one to five, the other twenty to twenty-four. Almost without hesitation she chose the fifth. She was about to show her collection on the fifth day of the fifth month, so said, 'Let's call it Number Five – I think it will bring me luck!' Little did she realise what luck she was about to unleash on herself and the world at large!

The secret of **No. 5**'s astounding success could be said to be partly in its packaging – the famous square bottle with its simple black-and-white label (the design has since entered the permanent collection at New York's Museum of Modern Art). Or it could be explained by its daring use of aldehydes, those synthetic smell-alikes which had been regarded with so much suspicion before the perfume's arrival. No. It is much simpler than that. It succeeded, and still does, because it is outspoken and completely unique. Nothing else smells like it, and nothing else would dare to! It's reported to contain a staggering 250 ingredients, but the ones that dominate are rose and jasmine. To this base is added ylang ylang, Dutch jonquil, Florentine iris, orange blossom, lily of the valley, mimosa, tonka bean, musk, patchouli, vetyver and sandalwood, all anchored in amber and civet. Balanced with aldehydes to give it its characteristic sheeny veneer, it finally becomes a totally harmonious blend that scintillates, insinuates and exudes sophistication. No wonder women love it, and men love smelling them in it!

What to wear it with, where and when

No. 5 is a perfume that's blissfully ignorant of the boundaries of age, convention, fashion or temperament. Not even colours or clothes matter much. The only thing that does is that you must complement its incomparable beauty and immense individuality. It has the enviable versatility of being able to be worn anywhere. Chanel herself mischievously advised that women should wear it 'wherever they want to be kissed!'

No. 19
by Chanel

*D*iscovering, rediscovering, or simply wearing **No. 19** is like entering an enchanted forest. Gabrielle Chanel regarded this as her very favourite perfume – the one that was named after her birthdate, 19 August, created initially for her private use and later given to her very favoured friends and valued clients. The rest of the world had to wait. That was before 1970, and when Chanel died in 1971, **No. 19** was released at large – I like to think in remembrance and honour of her. It was an instant sensation.

It's rare these days to find a perfume so totally bewitching as this. It's a beautiful ambery wood nymph. Consider its ingredients: **No. 19's** foresty, earthy pungency comes mostly from scented mosses, *fougère* (fern or bracken), bark, sandalwood, cedarwood and sycamore. Over this forest floor is scattered a handful of white hyacinth, Florentine iris, violet leaves and tenacious ylang ylang. Then to fix this fantasia for a long-lasting effect, musk and resinous amber are added.

The surprising thing about **No. 19** is that no one ingredient stands out from the others. It achieves a perfumed synergy that defies the usual analysis.

So let it remain a mystery with its golden brilliance, its dazzling, earthy warmness. Like a forest after rain, it shimmers and shines and haunts with its brooding beauty.

It's its own little universe of sunlight and shadow, of leaves fallen to earth and crushed underfoot, releasing a glowing and pulsating pungency. It has a wistful melancholy, a nostalgia that's utterly endearing. That's why **No. 19** is always such a pleasure to wear.

What to wear it with, where and when

Age first. **No. 19** is deliriously happy with the young but not terribly kind to anyone over forty, unless she still possesses youthful gusto. Colours should tend toward the earthy end of the spectrum, but reds and yellows and even white are okay, especially in crisp cotton. **No. 19** loves the likes of fine wool, alpaca, tweed, linen, cashmere and suede for day, and filmy chiffons and tulles by night. It also adores furs, faux or otherwise, but keep flashy jewellery away from it, and definitely no pearls! Although it particularly loves summer and autumn, this perfume has enough warmth to enliven even winter.

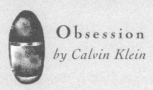

Obsession
by Calvin Klein

Obsession, being one of the vanguard of strong outspoken American perfumes, and also enormously
successful worldwide, has come in for more than its
fair share of flack. As a perfume it seems to be quite at odds
with the Calvin Klein look: it is anything but clean-cut,
pared-down or simple. Instead it's unashamedly sexy, brash
and sensual. It doesn't pretend to have subtle harmonies or
an interplay of notes that unfold gently to create an ever-
shifting emphasis and nuance. Instead it makes its point
quickly, definitely, unmistakably, with a strong clear note
that doesn't alter much with its duration on the skin.

Its main theme is amber – repeated over and over again.
It's above this constant melody that the other ingredients
are introduced, to merge with and intensify the amber
ambience. There are the rich floral presences of rose and
jasmine with plenty of orange blossom, a heady smell that is
quite simpatico with amber's persuasion. Then the mellow
end of the citrus brigade marches in with mandarin and
bergamot, followed by spicy coriander, French marigold and
oakmoss. It's all quite deliberately seductive, and fiercely
tenacious too, so don't be over-lavish with it.

Obsession is rather like a ground-to-air missile,
programmed to burst through any defence system to hit its

target. It's a perfume which is out to win, and does, one way or another, with its pounding pervasiveness, persistent sensuality, and unbridled suggestiveness. It certainly sums up the emotion it was named after.

What to wear it with, where and when

There's nothing to be gained from trying to marry the ultra-simple look of Klein's clothes to **Obsession**; it's far better served by sexier clothes – off-shoulder, halter-necked, bare-backed, mini, transparent, what have you. Stick to black and earthy colours, especially fiery orange, red and gold. If you must wear it with white make sure it doesn't look virginal or bridal. Big effects definitely work best. It's strictly 'evenings only', and only for the worldly and predatory. Lock it away from teens and grandmas.

Opium
by Yves Saint Laurent

PRONUNCIATION: eve-sarn-lor-ON

*Y*ves must have chuckled up his elegant sleeve when he heard that a peanut-growing Queensland premier had this perfume banned in his state. Perhaps he imagined it was habit-forming! In truth, **Opium** *has* had a narcotic effect on its users. Once sniffed, you can't keep away from it. Since its release in the seventies it has had a strong, one might even say addicted, group of supporters. And why not?

At the time of its arrival, oriental perfumes had been unfashionable for so long that women had either forgotten or never even encountered them. **Opium** changed that once and for all. Strangely, though, **Opium** is not a pure oriental type, being a lot lighter and more cosmopolitan than its darker-intentioned, kohl-eyed cousins like **Shalimar** and **Tabu**. Long before slick journalists used the word 'floriental' to describe an oriental with floral overtones, **Opium** had already combined these forces.

Its brilliant shimmer begins with a lush floral bouquet of jasmine and carnation. With this white splendour comes an invitation to enter the Garden of Allah: mandarin, patchouli, balsam, benzoin, frankincense, ginger, cinnamon, coriander, cedarwood and ylang ylang let off their brilliant fireworks! This wonderful salvo is vaulted into a dynamic airiness which threatens to explode, and indeed **Opium** is a perfume to be handled with care, or at least discretion.

It is a no-holds-barred adventure, poised, intoxicating and extremely sophisticated. It is a sheer tigress – invincible and fearless. No wonder it scared off a peanut farmer!

What to wear it with, where and when

Opium was born for blaze – gold, red, copper, silver, purple and lots of shiny black. It is most successful with slinky clothes and adores prowling around in silk, satin, brocade, jersey, velvet, sequins and beads, fabrics which lend themselves to the night and its seductive wiles. This perfume is not for the young or those who've missed the gravy train. Nor is it for the wives of peanut farmers – unless, of course, they're leaving the farm for worldlier pursuits.

Oscar de la Renta
by Oscar de la Renta

*P*erhaps only a Latin temperament could have carried off a perfume like **Oscar de la Renta** with such innate skill and casual ease. Like the man himself and the clothes he designs, this is a charming, refined and utterly dazzling little number. It aims directly for the glitzy life, its glossy edge barely concealing the *enfant sauvage* lurking just behind the cultivated orchids.

In the face of some pretty stiff opposition, this perfume has prospered mightily since its heady launch way back in 1977. Women never seem to tire of its powers of sweet seduction, its hypnotic Caribbean spell. To call it light is to deny its complexity. It is as luscious as a tropical breeze laden with jungle flowers, as lucid as a spectacular island dawn. It is this delicacy, this crystalline fragility, that Oscar de la Renta intended to capture. And he has, right down to the abstract flower-shaped stopper atop the beautifully curved bottle, with a dewdrop nestled in its glass petals.

The first whiff of the perfume is always a pleasure, bursting through with a barrage of flower scents so light they are almost impossible to identify. The core, elusive as it is, is that tropical charmer, ylang ylang, with top notes of tuberose, Bulgarian rose and jasmine. This is intensified even further with orange blossom and a glorious *bouquet garni* of herbs such as basil and coriander, then spiced with nutmeg and clove buds. A final veil of orientalism is laid over this garden of scents with sandalwood, opoponax (a sweet, warm resin), Moroccan myrrh and wisps of musk and vanilla. It's all an enticing enchantment, typical of the dazzling de la Renta style.

What to wear it with, where and when

Practically any colour suits the versatility of **Oscar de la Renta**, although browns, greys and navy might be a touch too stern for its extravagant flowering. It adores well-cut clothes of either classic elegance or flamboyant splendour. Day or night suits it well, with evening bringing out its seductiveness most eloquently. Its discreet charms and refined glamour melt even the hardest hearts, thus it likes all ages. Best of all, men love it. To them it is feminine without being fussy, elegant without being snooty and charming without being brash.

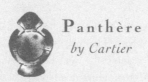

Panthère
by Cartier

PRONUNCIATION: parn-TAIR

KART-ee-air

*T*he House of Cartier is solidly synonymous with
la panthère couchée, or reclining panther. Now, to
reinforce its feline image, Cartier has named its
second perfume after this mysterious and powerfully beautiful animal.

Panthère as a perfume is probably not what you'd
expect. Instead of possessing a *femme fatale* savagery it is
instead extremely friendly and civilised, giving more of a
kittenish purr than a jungle snarl. But it is not without
considerable seductive powers; poised for the kill, **Panthère**
uses sophistication and allure as its weapons.

With a physique as sleek and muscular as its mascot's,
it launches its top notes with lots of heady tuberose,
jasmine, orange flowers and a hint of iris. From here we
enter the panther's warm, pulsating heart with a delicious
mix of tangerine, vetyver, patchouli, sandalwood and oakmoss, and dashes of nutmeg to spice things in readiness
for the passionate finale of civet, ambergris, musk,
opononax and a splash of beautiful Bourbon vanilla.
Surprisingly, all this makes for a most elegant and refined

pleasure, with fascinating depths and sparkling facets. Not the least imperious or overbearing, **Panthère**, despite its pedigree, has an understated opulence and an insistent sensuality. It doesn't leap out and attack but simply insinuates – stealthily. It is a very civilised prowler.

What to wear it with, where and when

This is a natural for all the gold, jet, ruby, tourmaline, topaz colours – anything blood-red or bronzed. Clothes should be very swish and dramatic – nothing frilly, tizzy or vulgar. And you can leave your casuals in the closet! **Panthère** is for the ultra-sophisticated huntress, so prettiness and niceness will get you nowhere. It needs a strong, sensual creature to wear it to the big occasions and ritzy parties it adores. It is a perfume that this particular type of woman will make her own. She will be poised and elegant but not over fifty. On her, **Panthère** is a killer.

Parfum d'été
by Kenzo

For anyone like myself pining for the heady days of **Vert et Blanc**, **Chypre**, **Emeraude**, **Réplique** and **Crêpe de Chine**, the great 'green' perfumes of the past, the name of this perfume sends out messages of hope. **Parfum d'été** – 'perfume of summer'. Despite this dreamy, pastoral name, **Parfum d'été** is not a pure greenie but a green-flavoured floral with curious oriental overtones. Be that as it may, it is still utterly delicious!

In making this perfume, Kenzo ('Japanese by birth, Parisian by chance') wanted to epitomise summer, to awaken all the senses to an impression of this exhilarating season. With typical Japanese poeticism he envisaged dawn, noon and dusk unfolding in sensuous rhythms, subtly changing with light and warmth. So, **Parfum d'été** is artfully composed to simulate the experience of passing through a summer's day.

The beginnings of this idyllic day are encapsulated in a haze of the scent of green sap and leaves, all tender and dewy, enmeshed with a secret flower that gently heralds the floral procession to follow. In the heightening warmth, flowers open to the sun, exuding their vibrating scents –

hyacinth and freesia for sweetness, narcissus and peony for piquancy, rose and jasmine for romance. Then, afternoon glides and fades into the enchantment of dusk with mysterious woodland calls of sandalwood, oakmoss and sun-warmed iris. With a discreet addition of musk and amber, Kenzo's summer's day is complete, but its languid sensuousness lingers on and on in a hush of nocturnal longing.

Parfum d'été is tranquil without being vague or amorphous. Its delicate subtlety is comforting and enveloping. And Kenzo, being a master of design, has contained his wondrous tribute to summer in a leaf-shaped, veined, frosted glass bottle. It epitomises, almost as much as the lovely perfume it holds, the breathtaking sparkle and light of the season of green delights.

What to wear it with, where and when

The greens have it here, and the pastels too. Since you wouldn't really bother to wear **Parfum d'été** in any other seasons but spring and summer, clothes should be light, diaphanous, feminine and ultra-simple in cotton, voile, chiffon, silk, georgette, lace and muslin. It's a knockout on lazy afternoons and at dusky twilight. Loving the outdoors, it doesn't care much for being cooped up at cocktail parties or the opera, though it might survive the ballet. Anyone from fourteen to a hundred can lose themselves in the midsummer dream of **Parfum d'été**, but it's best on blondes with green eyes and slightly freckled skins.

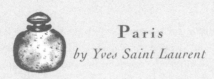

Paris
by Yves Saint Laurent

PRONUNCIATION: par-EE
eve sarn-lor-ON

*J*ust a whiff of this intoxicating tribute to the great city and it practically wafts you there on a magical breeze of rose petals and other luscious springtime blooms. For Saint Laurent, **Paris** is something of a bittersweet lament for the city as it was when he conquered it. Paris may have changed, but the rose still stalwartly remains the undoubted monarch that symbolises this city of fabulous colour, beauty and culture.

The first thing that surprised me about **Paris**, having already been told it was an intensely rosy perfume, was that although roses dominated the top notes, they certainly didn't reign alone. The very evident presence of violet came through so strongly I almost lost the roses for a while! The violets are there all the time, underscoring, but not competing. This means that **Paris** could never be described as a single-flower perfume, but more as a multi-floral based on roses. The exotic Arabian radiance of Damascus rose provides the initial heft, to be followed by a potpourri of other sweet and rare old-fashioned roses. Then the violets waft in, to be followed by a complex orchestration of mimosa, hyacinth, rose-scented geranium leaves, musk, sandalwood and cedar. All this makes for a spellbinding fugue, and a rather fortissimo one at that. There's nothing reticent about this **Paris**!

It's a joyous and brilliant perfume – very vivacious and laughing. It's one that romantic women love to have floating around them. **Paris** is like the sudden rush of love, new or renewed, expected or unexpected, that is so often inspired by the rose. It is Saint Laurent looking at Paris, perhaps at life itself, through rose-coloured glasses.

What to wear it with, where and when

Paris likes all colours. Wear it with anything beautiful, fresh, crisp or dazzling, either swathed or frilled or easily tailored. All ages smell ravishing in it, but especially the young and anyone in love. Day or night are equally fine for its rosy embrace, and seasons don't pose a particular problem either, although spring is obviously prime time for its floral overload. Occasions? Practically everything on the social calendar, but especially your birthday. **Paris** promises to take years off you!

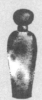

Pleasures
by Estée Lauder

PRONUNCIATION: ESS-tay LOR-da

Enter the newest member of the formidable Lauder line-up, a perfume that is exactly what its name suggests.

Pleasures is a totally new departure for Lauder. It's quite undramatic, undemonstrative and understated. It also has the distinction of totally ignoring the current plethora of 'fruit salad' fragrances by resolutely sticking to flowers – and more flowers! I like it almost without reservation for its openness, its vivacity and its sheer *joie de vivre*!

It's called a 'sheer' perfume, meaning transparent, but its formulation is conversely complex. With its pretty bouquet of white lilies and violet leaves accented with fresh greenery, it has a winning innocence right from the start. Once its top notes are established, the middle ones creep in to consolidate the floral impression with darker lilies (said to be black), white peonies (very delicate and slightly spicy), pink roses and lots of natural jasmine to add a little voluptuousness to the proceedings. Then a most fascinating note of Baie Rose underscores all this with its warm, peppery smell, and the whole gorgeous bouquet is rounded out with some sandalwood and patchouli to keep the scent lingering.

To me, **Pleasures** smells like a garden after rain — fresh, intense and piquant. It is sweet without being cloying, romantic without being soppy, soft but clear and high-singing. Best of all, for Lauder devotees it fills the gap between the outright sumptuousness of **Beautiful** and the scrubbed-clean simplicity of **White Linen**. **Pleasures** is a pretty but sensible young thing that values its innocence. That's what makes it so tantalising.

What to wear it with, where and when

For sweet sixteens to bittersweet thirties, this is a perfume for the young. Clothes that are young and adventurous are perfect for it. It loves fresh colours, but only at the soft end of the spectrum. Go for white, pink, pale blues and greens, mauve, lavender, lemon and apricot in billowy fabrics like chiffon, silk, georgette or the crispness of cotton and piqué. You can wear denim if you like, but don't expect the perfume to smell quite as charmingly innocent. **Pleasures** complements most occasions with gentle ease, but doesn't care much for sports or dressed-up gatherings. Come spring and summer it is in seventh heaven.

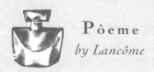

Pôeme
by Lancôme

The current Lancôme catalogue of perfumes is beautifully balanced with the much-loved **Trésor**, the seductively beautiful **Magie Noir** and the stunningly cool **Ô de Lancôme**. So its newest, **Pôeme**, has a pretty hard act to follow. But it lives up to the reputation of its sister perfumes with typical Lancôme grace and ease.

Created by a great French nose named Jacques Cavallier, **Pôeme** is composed entirely of flowers, which is unusual, since very few perfumes today can honestly claim to be completely floral. It is also linked, like all things poetic, to a Muse. The French actress Juliette Binoche, a latter-day gamine but one possessed of truly radiant and charming contradictions, was chosen by Lancôme to epitomise its perfume with her mercurial magnetism.

So what of the resulting perfume itself? It begins with an unexpected harmony of two opposing types of flowers – the seductive, carnal scent of the *Datura candida*, a desert flower, and the blue poppy, a rare flower from the Himalayas. This has a scent so delicate it is quite impossible to use naturally, so its mountain-air freshness and luminosity is replicated in the laboratory. Added to these rare beauties is a bouquet of sunlit yellow flowers – freesia, roses and mimosa – and the opulent white flowers of the vanilla vine.

Inasmuch as any perfume can claim to be liquid poetry, **Pôeme** is. It uniquely expresses the subliminal intensity of poetry translated into the lyricism and sensuality representative of a woman. The result is a perfume that speaks yearningly of love and adoration. It is not an epic ode to perfume but an enticing vision of what a woman may need to express her own rapturous and romantic individuality.

What to wear it with, where and when

Pôeme is a very extroverted perfume and needs bright or vibrant colours to bring out its best – reds, blues, oranges and yellows. Black is okay, but white is better. Clothes should be chic, whether they're casual or dressy. Don't wear anything tizzy or frothy – **Pôeme** is too refined for nonsense. Fabrics can be anything from cotton to satin, but no roughies like denim. I'd keep it for semi-formal to formal occasions, as well as at home or in the office. Seasons don't bother it, and as for age, like all good poetry it spans the years with ease, appealing to the sensitive woman no matter if she's twenty or eighty.

Poison
by Christian Dior

PRONUNCIATION: PWAH-son or POY-zun

Shrieks of surprise, derision and sheer disbelief echoed through the perfume industry when the House of Dior launched its radical new perfume in 1985. The project had been under wraps for three years and everyone knew something revolutionary was about to be detonated, but no one could believe their astonished ears when it was finally unveiled in a barrage of blazing publicity – **Poison**!

The new stance taken by Dior upset the sacrosanct applecart, leading to other blockbusters like **Dune** and **Fahrenheit**. People were shocked that such a respectable house would have the gall to call a perfume by such a name. But, after a good decade or so, the visionaries at Dior proved themselves right. For, like it or loathe it, **Poison** has stood its ground.

As a perfume it is utterly unique – still! In creating it, perfumer Edouard Flechler rejected the usual floral bouquet springboard and based his idea on a highly original opening accord of spices and herbs. **Poison**'s initial clout comes from a daring combination of Russian coriander and Ceylonese cinnamon. This is the radical departure point for a potion which, along the way, also adds berries, pepper, grape and exotic fruits for a volcanic eruption before softening the aftermath with a forthright dash of sumptuous roses and sexy vanilla. The result is *not* pretty, romantic or even particularly charming. Instead it is downright audacious!

Poison is very much a perfume of the liberated woman – independent, assertive, uncompromising, dauntless. Whether its name implies witchcraft, lethal spells or worse is neither here nor there. It is its own weapon, with an explosive impact as unflinching as its marvellous purple bottle. If you're the right woman for its dynamism, you'll make some memorable entrances and even more dramatic exits.

What to wear it with, where and when

It's absolutely fabulous with rich purple, violet, heliotrope, cerise, scarlet, crimson, vermilion, shocking pink, gold, silver and, best of all, black! It loves expensive *anything*, particularly exotic jewellery (tons of it) and fabulous furs. It just adores being dressed to kill. Sinister on the elderly, laughable on the young, it is strictly the domain of the self-assured, sophisticated mature woman with more than her fair share of brains and beauty. All seasons are fine with it, particularly winter nights when it glows like an exotic jewel.

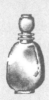

Private Collection
by Estée Lauder

PRONUNCIATION: ESS-tay LOR-da

*K*nown to be a woman of formidable taste, Estée Lauder for years dressed herself in a perfume that became her signature – an accessory synonymous with her elegant image. Naturally she had it created wholly and solely for her use, to her own formulation. But two women – the Duchess of Windsor and Princess Grace of Monaco – admired it so much she gave it to them as an exclusive present. Finally, after their passings, she released the precious perfume to the world at large and called it, naturally enough, **Private Collection**. It was to be a perfume worn when you wanted people to say, in fascinated wonderment, 'Who *is* that woman?'

On the right woman **Private Collection** is indeed a disturbing and eloquent perfume. It exudes an enormous self-confidence with a polished patina of well-bred luxury and elegance. The perfume is described by Lauder as a floral blend, but I would tend to put it into a much greener category. Whilst not being a true green, it has a decidedly leafy, grassy presence that pervades its considerably lush garden of flowers: Bulgarian rose, orange flower, jasmine, heliotrope, and chrysanthemum. The greenery comes from linden blossom and sappy green leaves (probably galbanum) and the gently insistent sandalwood. It all amounts to a carefully harmonised graciousness – not flamboyant, but exquisite and pervasive without actually achieving any great depth or complexity.

Private Collection is meant to be noticed and noted in polite social circles. It adds a personal aura of serene aloofness, with a surface friendliness that is quite detached from things and people beneath it. No wonder Mrs Lauder made it her own!

What to wear it with, where and when

Think of the New York upper crust, the café society, the rich and the famous, and you've got the message of **Private Collection**. Subtle, classy colours like rich cream, ivory, coffee, pearl grey, silver, amethyst, garnet and tourmaline are its counterpoint, with discreet flashes of rose gold. Clothes must be extremely well-tailored and under-decorated. Wool jersey, velvet, silk, lace, crêpe and chiffon are the go. This perfume revels in social circles where guests have been carefully selected for their charm, availability and/or money. Being witty helps too. Certainly never to be worn out of doors in any season, and not to be touched by anyone under thirty.

Red
by Giorgio Beverly Hills

*I*n its vibrant red packaging and tall, statuesque bottle, Giorgio's **Red** is strident! Assertive, complex, definite and defiant, it's one of those perfumes with the questionable tendency to walk ahead of its wearer (though perhaps not *quite* so far as its predecessor, **Giorgio**).

Despite its emphatic attitude, **Red** has a certain subtlety of spirit, probably because its formula boasts no fewer than 692 ingredients, so we are told! Its initial notes are heady flower essences – mainly carnation and jasmine – with the mesmeric rareness of osmanthus to give a soft oriental diffusion. Then fruits are added, along with dazzling dashes of nutmeg and clove for a pungent spike. The lovely chypre procession then enters with gently pervasive oakmoss over green leaves and grassy notes, all cloaked in liquid amber. This has the effect of giving a fresh piquancy and sharpness that glides leisurely into the more feminine, rounded middle notes. Gradually a soft but tenacious finale is achieved quite deftly with a fruit and vanilla fade-out that's lingering without overstaying its welcome.

Red is not a pretty perfume, nor an especially romantic one. It means business in no uncertain terms. It makes its point definitely but politely and, once made, sparkles and twitters quite charmingly as it floats through its own orbit.

Even though its publicists boast that no one should ever underestimate the power of a woman in **Red**, it's not really theatening at all. The woman attracted to it will not be a power-crazed monster sweeping all before her. She'll be a clever, witty, urbane creature, and quite level-headed too – a woman who seduces charmingly without playing the heavy.

What to wear it with, where and when

Red handles all the shades and intensities of its namesake, plus black, white, silver and gold. Warm earthy tones don't suit its urbanity, and pastels shrink from its bravado. It can manage night or day equally well, dressed in that hard-edged, pared-down American simplicity. It may be a touch too obvious for the office, and far too pushy for the boudoir, but otherwise it's socially polite and malleable. It's not for the young or the old, being more in the sights of the career girl. It is a woman's weapon, but far from lethal – just a little dangerous.

Red Door
by Elizabeth Arden

The entrances to the hallowed sanctuaries of Elizabeth Arden Beauty Salons have always been distinguished by their elegantly panelled pillarbox red portals. Behind these discreet doors, millions of women have surrendered their bodies and souls to the pampering attentions of the Arden beauticians, partaking of those mysterious rituals that usually culminate in a fragrant flourish of the current number one Arden perfume. Today a woman would probably be wreathed in a spray of **Red Door**, the House's most successful perfume.

This is Arden's tribute to the modern woman. **Red Door** is very popular, with a high social profile and a cool self-confidence. It is unselfconsciously assertive, having no soft edges but a rather aggressive attitude under its outward show of femininity. It assumes the mantle of sophistication without actually being all that sophisticated. To put it bluntly, **Red Door** champions the go-ahead woman, pushing her forward so she doesn't get lost in the background.

Its formulation is a complicated affair with an intensely floral approach that's not in the least softly-lit or seductive. Its florals are highly glamorous, a haughty mix dominated by three powerful scents – tea rose, freesia and the elusive *Cymbidium karan*, an orchid so rarefied it blooms only briefly in winter under strictly controlled conditions. Backing up these scents are fairly ferocious sweeps of ylang ylang, wild violet, jasmine, lily of the valley, and Moroccan orange blossom. Further back there's also an undertone of honeysuckle, the sharp green of vetyver and a softening hush of sandalwood. It adds up to a collective clout known in perfume circles as 'ultra-modern'.

Red Door does what it sets out to do most successfully. It always guarantees a presence that is confident and uplifting. It is no shy retiring violet.

What to wear it with, where and when

Red Door is a creature of the concrete jungle, with its kaleidoscopic dazzle and energy, so forget about featuring it on picnics and the like. Keep it for town and for the evening, wearing it with red, black or any of the intense earth colours. It won't really hold its own on big occasions, but in lesser social situations it fares quite well, as long as you can match its brilliance and self-assurance. Not good on the young, and too hard-edged for the elderly, it's best on the mature woman of some poise. It's also trans-seasonal, but I wouldn't wear it in a heatwave.

Rive Gauche
by Yves Saint Laurent

PRONUNCIATION: HREEV-goash
eve sarn lor-ON

*I*f ever there was a perfect 'desert island' perfume, this cheeky charmer would be it! If some terrible calamity befell one, and one had the chance of taking a single perfume to mythical isolation, this ageless, seasonless, insouciant *coquette* could be the one.

Saint Laurent's chameleon creation seems to cover just about every given situation, and complement every turn of temperament. It will blithely cope with any adventure or misadventure, and come smiling through. **Rive Gauche** has that rare capacity of smelling good on just about everyone.

When it was launched in 1971, Saint Laurent named **Rive Gauche** not so much for the racy left bank of Paris, but for his *prêt-à-porter* boutiques of the same name. It was one of the new-breed of 'moderns' to marry green aldehydic notes with a traditional floral bouquet, thus achieving a sharp and assertive difference.

Its bright top notes shoot off a barrage of jasmine, honeysuckle, narcissus, gardenia and green rose blended with other green notes of oakmoss, vetyver and galbanum, then underscored with orris root and sandalwood. This gives

Rive Gauche its sensuous and sexy middle and bottom tonalities. It's a stunning accord, distinctive and dazzling but not the least trashy or vulgar.

Rive Gauche has a restless energy, an upbeat *élan* all of its own. Bravado is its strong point, with a touch of mischief at the edges, but it would never bother to pretend to be anything but itself. Although the young may assume it to be their sole territory, more mature women can be flattered by its very youthfulness.

What to wear it with, where and when

After the above, it would seem pretty obvious that **Rive Gauche** is just dandy all year round, any time of day or night. As far as moods go it's a great cheer-up tonic, and dotes on noisy gatherings of all sorts, but it's also able to behave itself at more well-mannered gatherings, albeit with a sly wink. It likes over-the-top clothes in a riot of colour, but it's really more at home with terrific casuals and unconventional gear. It loves sport, outdoors or in, as long as it's on the move!

Romeo di Romeo Gigli

by Romeo Gigli

**PRONUNCIATION: rro-MAY-o
JEE-lee**

To Juliet's plaintive inquiry, 'O Romeo, Romeo where-fore art thou?', one could well reply, 'In this fantastic bottle, my love!' Like a medieval cone-shaped hat, **Romeo di Romeo Gigli**'s bottle is topped with a fanciful flourish of frosted glass like banners waving. But it's what's inside that's truly romantic.

Its exotic ingredients take you on a fabulous journey to the most romantic places on earth. With a sparkling prelude, **Romeo di Romeo Gigli** sets sail with citrus notes of Italian bergamot, mandarin, orange and lime. Then there's a whiff of basil from the Seychelles, golden African marigolds and Persian galbanum, together with blackcurrant and whimsical whiffs of lush Indian mango. Hard on the heels of this head-reeling introduction come great trumpetings of flowers, two of which come to dominate and give the perfume its unmistakable signature – 'living' freesia, and lily of the valley. The 'living' bit claims that an extraction process preserves the very essence of the flower with fidelity. I must say the freesia does smell startlingly lifelike, but happily it does not override the scent of the delicate lily.

There are more flowers to follow, though. On comes the sunny brightness of Spanish broom, heady Formosan orange blossom, rich Moroccan rose, Egyptian jasmine and French carnation. All of this is softened with a background allure of Arabian incense, Mysore sandalwood, Sumatran benzoin and the woody-violet hush of Florentine iris.

Romeo di Romeo Gigli is an incredibly intoxicating love potion — a luscious intertwining that sends out tantalising wafts of breezy sensuality. If you're in the least bit the dreamy or romantic type, you'll be a pushover for its charms. One can well imagine the love-mad Romeo totally succumbing to his sweet Juliet on her balcony if she sent out powerful love messages like this!

What to wear it with, where and when

Naturally you'd think of all the gossamer-light diaphanous fabrics in pale, shimmering colours, and that's certainly the story. Hard, dominating colours are competely alien to **Romeo**'s startstruck orbit, as is anything outdoorsy or energetic. It's a perfume created for the young and innocent, but it's not off-limits to career-movers and hard-edged sophisticates. It can hold its own practically anywhere, but may get lost in a crowd, so keep it for smaller and more intimate occasions. Wear it in spring and summer, when its delicacy sings with happiness.

Safari
by Ralph Lauren

*O*ne needn't be so slavish as to drag this perfume around in a Louis Vuitton haversack on an actual safari, but treat it rather as an elegant adjunct on one's journey through the great safari of life!

That's apparently how Mr Lauren hoped **Safari** would be regarded when he released it to his vast clientele of women. As an adventure in perfume it is not all that fearless or daring, and certainly not dangerous, but happily on the safe and sound side. It's a very congenial and gregarious perfume that hints at the wild rather than taking a game swipe at it up-front. **Safari** is refined, ladylike and good-natured.

Its basic structure is a medley of flowers and fruit with green and woody underpinnings. It begins with a burst of bright orange and blackcurrant bud backed with the sweet sharpness of jonquil and the softness of hyacinth. To these are added the indispensible *rose de mai* and jasmine, a hint of violet-like orris root, and more than a passing whiff of heady orange blossom.

Then the real heavies come in to give **Safari** its outdoors atmosphere. Apart from woods of sandal and cedar, there's a tenacious note of green vetyver, that wonderfully pungent oriental grass that enlivens many a perfume. It gives **Safari** an earthy greenness that accents all the highly scented flowers. The whole sojourn is rounded out with an admirably restrained dash of patchouli and some soothing amber to settle down the excitement to a reasonably low roar.

So, if armchair adventure is your idea of roughing it in the wild, **Safari** will set you happily dreaming of wide open spaces, sunny vistas and wild animals at a safe distance. If, however, you're after the hands-on thing, it could prove to be more of a hindrance than a help when that elephant comes trumpeting out of the jungle!

What to wear it with, where and when

Safari was created for comfort, but *elegant* comfort, in the style of most of Mr Lauren's clothes. Pants, anything that swings freely, classy casuals, well-cut denims and resort clothes are the go. All the earthy colours are tops with it, so put away the purples, pinks, greens and blues. As for occasions, it's out of place at glamorous gatherings, but daytime dalliances like shopping, visiting, lunching – and even a touch of love in the afternoon – are perfect. **Safari** doesn't care much for winter, but dotes on warmer weather. Age is unimportant as long as you've got a sense of adventure.

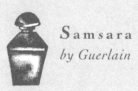

Samsara
by Guerlain

*H*eaven only knows how some great perfumes are born, but there are two versions of the birth of **Samsara**. One is that Jean Paul Guerlain went on a secret sojourn to India for a possible inspiration, and found it in the idea of combining large concentrations of Indian jasmine and sandalwood. The other is that he asked a very dear lady friend what she would like to smell in a new perfume. She said jasmine and sandalwood. Whichever is true, that's what his new perfume was eventually composed of. He then gave it the Sanskrit name of **Samsara** and unveiled his creation to the world.

It wasn't what most people expected, but it charmed everyone from the outset. Already it's been hailed as a classic, or at least one in the making. Its main claim to fame is its staggering content of sandalwood – 22 per cent essence, an extraordinary amount of such a precious ingredient. Properly balanced, as it is in **Samsara**, with loads of rich, creamy jasmine, it takes on a new bloom – a radiant resonance like a fine old viola rather than a highly strung violin. Added to this are deft touches of narcissus for a slightly sharper counterpoint, violet leaves, some roses, a good dash of bergamot and a twist of lemon. Finally, it is warmed with amber and finished off with the flourish of Guerlain's aphrodisiacal trademark, vanilla.

Samsara is without doubt a fabulously beautiful perfume, one with exquisite poise and polish. It spins in a heavenly orbit, softly, intriguingly, gradually luring you forward into its depths. Once there, you're caught in its intricate and beautiful web. And even after its discreet exit, which it makes without your being aware of it, the memory of it lingers in your head quite intoxicatingly – the sign of a very great perfume.

What to wear it with, where and when

Samsara is one of those rarities – a perfume that, if worn on the right woman at the right time, is indifferent to colours, textures and styles. Nevertheless it reveals itself most charmingly with sea greens and blues, and all the colours of a coral island – sand, sage, hibiscus, amber, and pale aquatic shades. It also adores cream, black, red and gold. It is wonderful with flowing fabrics and shines both day and night in spring and summer with its luminosity. Treat **Samsara** as you would a precious and rare flower – with deference and love. It will serve you eternally.

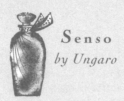

Senso
by Ungaro

PRONUNCIATION: oon-GAR-o

Senso is the baby of Ungaro's trio of perfumes. Joining the divine **Diva** and the uninhibited **Ungaro**, **Senso** is a lively and lyrical perfume. One look at its sensational packaging will tell you that. It comes in a statuesque shocking pink bottle, resembling fabric draped over a torso, and is finished with a brilliant yellow bow of black polka dots topped with a dazzling sapphire blue stopper. Very sassy, very Ungaro.

The perfume is not the heavy, sensual potion you might expect from its name. Its sensuality is more playful, full of luscious ripe fruit smells and heady flowers with an exotic slant. You may even detect the scent of apple lurking in the lush orchard, but the principal top notes are orange blossom and ylang ylang, both of them highly vibrant and intoxicating. Around these two beauties are the sun-dappled fruit harmonies tinged with zingy green.

Thus **Senso** has a remarkable zest and sparkle. It is dynamic and very extroverted – even cheeky! Its freshness is infectious, giving it an unbridled abandon and youthfulness.

Ungaro summarises the **Senso** woman as 'above all, sensuous . . . in matters of the heart she makes her own rules – and breaks them at will.' I can see his point. It is a mischievous perfume, capricious but with a secret strategy of ultimate seduction. You should have plenty of not-so-innocent fun with **Senso** to back you up!

What to wear it with, where and when

There's no use hiding your light under a bushel with **Senso**. Its brightness and vivacity positively scream for chirpy, jaunty colours in clothes that can be either devastatingly daring or cheekily *outré*. Avoid the heavies – no purple, black or grey – but choose brilliant reds and blues, yellows, greens and anything metallic and sparkly. Spring and summer are **Senso**'s blooming seasons, so the right stuff will be light and filmy – cottons, voiles, linens and chiffons. Day or night makes no difference to it, but I'm afraid if you're seriously over thirty you're on shaky ground!

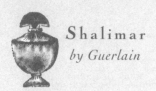

Shalimar
by Guerlain

PRONUNCIATION: SHALL-ee-mah
gair-LARN

Shalimar – surely the most beautiful word in all perfume. It's a word that insinuates with the sheer sensuousness of its sound, conjuring up the fabled fantasies of '1001 Nights' and the sight of the Taj Mahal in moonlight – a word that reverberates and haunts long after its sound has evaporated. It's the perfect name for a perfume steeped in oriental enigmas.

Created in 1925, **Shalimar** was designed to be overtly oriental. A certain chemist by the name of Justin Dupin had intrigued Jacques Guerlain with a new synthetic ingredient called vanillin. Although very similar to the vanilla bean-pod in smell, it actually came from a conifer sap derivative and smelled more like vanilla than vanilla itself. Grandfather Jacques had always been convinced that vanilla was a powerful aphrodisiac – a prerequisite of orientalia. He forthwith took some of his sensationally popular creation, **Jicky**, a revolutionary mix of herbs, citrus and lavender, added a generous dash of the upstart vanillin, plus sandalwood, spices, incense and the heady opoponax, and *voilà*! **Shalimar** was born. He put it in a magnificent

Baccarat bottle and it catapulted to instant stardom, becoming *the* quintessential oriental perfume.

Named after the Gardens of Shalimar in Lahore, India, which were created by the love-sick Shah Jehan in memory of his favourite wife Mumtaz Mahal (for whom the great Taj Mahal was built), **Shalimar** is a haunting tribute to woman's eternal love and beauty. It is a fabulous marvel – a langorous, piercingly sweet and nostalgic perfume. Just to utter its name is to be spellbound by it.

What to wear it with, where and when

Sorry, but if you're not sophisticated, witty, seductive and incurably romantic, forget the fireworks of **Shalimar**. Naturally it's not for the young, but the mature can revel in it because it has that rare ability to flatter and reveal a woman's aura of fascination. It's a great seducer and demands clothes and colours of intense persuasion with a hint of extravagance. Since **Shalimar** emanates a jewelled glitter, richly dark reds, serene purples and indigo, mysterious emerald colours and amethyst, topaz and tourmaline are its territory – nothing wishy-washy. This is an aristocrat to wear with sumptuous silks and satins, brocades and velvets, laces and furs. It also loves nocturnal intimacy and passion, and is best in autumn and winter, or any time when outright secuction is in the air.

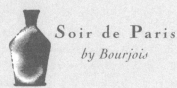

Soir de Paris
by Bourjois

PRONUNCIATION: swar duh par-EE
boure-ZJHWAH

*I*f you're old enough to remember the famous midnight blue bottle with the silver **Evening in Paris** label and you thought it was just a memory never to be sighted again, good news! **Soir de Paris** is back, still resplendent in its midnight blue Art Deco bottle.

The perfume has survived the comeback very well indeed. A mature lady of my acquaintance recently rediscovered it with girlish squeals of delight and said it hadn't changed a bit! Whether age has dimmed her memory or not I am too kind to conjecture, but it is a beguiling and enchanting perfume just the same.

Soir de Paris was created by the master perfumer of the twenties, Ernest Beaux, the genius who conjured up the redoubtable **No. 5** of Chanel. Need I say more! On its creation Monsieur Bourjois himself, obviously an astute entrepreneur, found an unprecedented way to promote his new perfume. Because sound movies had just hit Paris, he chose a theatre on the Champs Elysees and sprayed it with his precious perfume before each show! The ladies lapped it up and **Soir de Paris** became a roaring success.

Composed of light florals dashed with intriguing spices, **Soir de Paris** has an immediate feminine appeal that broadens out to reveal lovely subtleties. The top notes are enchanting violet with a touch of heliotrope, sweet pea and the green coolness of linden blossom. These are poised over a softly spiced base of vetyver, amber and incense, which mellows to a powdery delicacy and a bewitching fade-out. It's a perfume that lingers with an unobtrusive lightness and a poignant charm.

I, for one, am very glad it's back.

What to wear it with, where and when

My friend who wore **Soir de Paris** in her heyday was given to chic, sharply tailored little navy suits with white piqué trims and pleated and draped dresses of satin. I can see no reason why such style doesn't still hold for today's convert. Its delicacy loves pastels of blue, grey, green and (at a pinch) pink, but it's equally lovely with indigo, cobalt, powder blue, dusty rose, grey and black. **Soir de Paris** works beautifully with linen, wool, chiffon, silk and satin, but don't insult it with sporty denims, bright synthetics and the like. As to age, any woman with charm and a romantic bent can wear it well. It floats beautifully on the air in spring and summer.

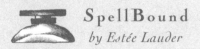

SpellBound
by Estée Lauder

This salvo, fired by the redoubtable Mrs Lauder, manages to be worlds away from the other Lauder perfumes by positioning itself in the so-called 'floriental' contingent. In other words, it has pretty equal proportions of flowers and spices.

SpellBound contains a great many things, but one of the most important and unusual is carnation, with its unique floral-clove scent. It adds to the overall complexity of the perfume, lingering in the air after the dominant jasmine and orange flower scents have succumbed to all the other flowers in this generous bouquet. These are gardenia, lily of the valley, rose and tuberose, with an edging of narcissus. Fruits also get a good look-in, with apricot, bergamot, peach and blackcurrant, before the really big oriental guns are brought in: vetyver, musk, amber, cinnamon, clove, sandalwood and a powerful dash of vanilla bean. The effect is more emphatic than mysterious, but certainly mesmerising.

SpellBound doesn't weave a spell – it hurls it out as a challenge. It's very forthright, out to seduce with no thought of time-wasting foreplay. But it's not cold and calculating, having an overt warmth that is disturbing and magnetic. It's like being stroked with long velvet gloves: its strategy of conquest is not subtle, but a foregone conclusion.

What to wear it with, where and when

SpellBound favours the dark end of the colour spectrum – black, parma violet, umber and chocolate, along with outspoken blood red, orange, magenta and gold. It's great with the heavier fabrics – velvet, wool, cashmere, fur, leather, suede. Filmy things seem uncomfortable in its relentless presence. It's a highly sexed fragrance and goes with anything tight and clinging, including body-hugging jeans and leather jackets worn with studded pants. For evening, dramatic, low-cut numbers are naturals. It's too dangerous for the young, but if you're in any way wild or wanton, **SpellBound** will do wonders for you. But don't drench yourself in it. Too much and you'll break the spell.

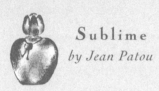

Sublime
by Jean Patou

Since the death of Patou (one of the most elegantly influential of all Parisian *couturièrs*) only one perfume has emerged from the House of Patou – the magnificently grand **1000**. Now comes **Sublime**, bearing absolutely no resemblance to its predeccessor. In fact, it is a rather surprising entry into a market bursting at the seams with assertive, strident perfumes, all desperate for attention. I doubt if **Sublime** has made more than a ripple on the olfactory pond – it is certainly not a perfume that trumpets its attributes from the rooftops. What I'm saying is, don't expect a perfume that will knock your head off. But *do* expect a most exquisite, subtle and joyous perfume.

Sublime is actually a resurrection of a lovely but long-gone beauty by Patou, called **Colony**. Made just before World War II, this perfume featured daring notes of pineapple and ylang ylang. **Sublime** uses the same fruit and flower accord, but this time with the emphasis on citrus fruits. It begins with a dazzling display of hypnotic ylang ylang underscoring Sicilian orange and mandarin, and then floats them into a lovely mix of lily of the valley, orange blossom, rose and jasmine with hints of green oakmoss, vetyver and soft sandalwood. All this is then secured with a sturdy vanilla base note, giving off a powdery diffusion.

There's absolutely nothing emphatic or outspoken about **Sublime**. Its manners are refined, poised and sensual in the tender sense. It's a perfume that has a glorious radiance, a tranquil intimacy that always reminds me of Grand Marnier sipped slowly at sunset.

What to wear it with, where and when

Sublime positively radiates its gentle warmth in yellows and oranges, and gives a healthy kick to beige, brown and red. It's not a great lover of the outdoors, preferring to weave its spell at intimate dinners and sophisticated gatherings. If you're off to gape at the Louvre or go first-nighting to the Paris Opera, **Sublime** is bliss. Its cultivated subtlety needs very beautiful clothes. If you're the madly extroverted type, forget it. And if you're very young you probably won't find it action-packed or glittery enough either. But if you are over twenty and can muster up moods of elegant calm and natural poise, its discreet but stylish panache will enhance your radiance.

Tabu
by Dana

Before you incredulously screech '*Tabu*?!', let me remind you that this much-maligned perfume has been around the traps since 1930, so it's obviously got something going for it. For more than sixty years, **Tabu** has remained faithful to its following with nary an alteration to its formula or its promotional image. The famous ad in which a male violinist sweeps a crinolined pianist off her stool with a passionate kiss, announcing **Tabu** as 'the forbidden perfume', still gets the same message across with a dramatic flourish.

These days it's more likely to turn up on supermarket shelves than in perfume boutiques. It's amazingly inexpensive, but those who loftily poo-poo it as cheap are snobs, as far as I'm concerned. If you like it, wear it, especially if it likes you! **Tabu** was always noted for its potency, but at least you don't have to literally scrub it off like some of its modern rivals. Just the same, I'd advise that you be discreet with it to be on the safe side.

Tabu is a straight-out, hands-on, no-holds-barred oriental of quite awesome power. It blends the usual jasmine and rose, but with substantial buffers of patchouli, orange flower, bergamot, clove bud, oakmoss and various mystery spices, and fixes the whole highly inflammable cocktail with nothing less than the devastating animal note of civet. There's no escaping it!

Of course, **Tabu** is not a perfume to be toyed with. Definitely R-rated, on some unsuspecting skins it becomes practically X-rated! It radiates its sexuality with extraordinary disregard to subtlety. It's a bit like that scene in *The Barefoot Contessa* where Ava Gardner kicks off her stilettos and whips up a storm in a gypsy camp with a very camp Apache-cum-flamenco dance. And when the dust settles, that's where **Tabu** steps in to complete the kill. It may not be refined, but boy, it's got guts!

What to wear it with, where and when

You might gather from the above that wearing anything remotely Laura Ashley is out of the question with **Tabu**. This is strictly torrid territory, with a *femme fatale* look that's slightly rough at the edges. Anything that smacks of smoulder is a must: black, red, all the hot Spanish colours, in clothes that do most of the work for you without the fuss of frills. Not for the young and uninitiated, it's strictly for the worldly, sensuous woman with the gypsy in her soul and a fair whack of desire up front. Seasons are immaterial to its powers, but I think it's best left for after-dark occasions. It is, of course, absolutely incendiary in the boudoir, being born of the bordello.

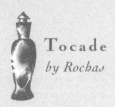

Tocade
by Rochas

PRONUNCIATION: tock-ARD
hro-SHAR

Translation? Take your pick from 'love at first sight', 'infatuation', or 'a strong and sometimes unreasonable attraction'. Rochas's latest addition to its formidable repertoire of classy perfumes is, like all its others, intensely feminine and unmistakably French. It's a perfume full of light, romance and radiance.

Tocade is described as being like a performance in three acts. The curtain rises on a rush of rose given a bolstering with orange-scented bergamot, then quickly engaged to heady magnolia blossoms and tangy geranium before the sudden dramatic entrance of vanilla in all its sensual creaminess and suggestiveness. Quite a plot unravelling! Act two is where the complications set in, with denser, more serious notes of seductive Turkish rose, another shot of vanilla to keep the plot thickening, then rich notes of cedar, rare amber and benzoin (a chocolaty vanilla-drenched resin). Act three rounds off the performance, gathering the cast happily together and cementing the relationships with a soft, powdery veil of musk and more amber. The curtain falls on a happy ending.

All this luscious radiance is then poured into glass bottles of bright jewel-like colours, so attractive that, in the words of one witty scribe, 'It's a toss-up between the bottle and the contents!'

As a perfume it is neither strident nor demanding, yet it's a good deal more subtle and manipulative than you might first imagine, so don't pass judgment too quickly by thinking it's just another light, flowery-fruity cocktail. It's much more sophisticated and insistent than that.

If you're the open-hearted, impetuous type that falls in love all too easily, beware **Tocade** – its intoxicating message might involve you in more serious matters of the heart than you bargained for.

What to wear it with, where and when

The nicest thing about **Tocade** is its friendliness: it couldn't care less whether you're eighteen or eighty, poor or rich, frilly or discreet. It graces all with its good-natured charm and exuberance. Thus it revels in pastels, neutrals and vibrants, as well as being a knockout in white. Any frou-frou you like to whip up is fine, and it adores ultra-feminine, unashamedly romantic clothes. Although it prefers carefree events, it can manage enough chic for a cocktail bash. Seasons don't worry it much, but I'd give it a rest in winter.

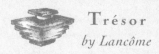

Trésor
by Lancôme

a rose by any other name *does* smell as sweet, and in this case, the name of the rose is **Trésor**. It is the inspiration, the heart and the point of departure for this fascinatingly different perfume.

Unfortunately, **Trésor** is one of those perfumes that seems to polarise women. Some are utterly devoted to it, others dislike it intensely. I think the reason for one's liking it or not rests with its soft sweetness, its very powdery pervasiveness. There's not a sharp, let alone shrill, note in its make-up, which is understandable when you consider its rosy heart, its lavish bouquet of lilac, iris and heliotrope with a slight spring dash of lily of the valley and, I suspect, a hint of violet. Then there's the delicious addition of ripe peach and golden apricot over a beautifully balanced base of sandalwood, amber, musk and vanilla.

Admittedly, all this has a certain confectionery quality about it, an old-fashioned sentimentality that might stick in the craw of the less romantically inclined. But I find it a pleasure and something of a surprise that a relatively new perfume can have such good manners and feminine grace –

a quiet and dignified beauty that ignores passing fads to create its own distinctive world.

Trésor is not a perfume that grabs you in a vice, demanding to be tried. It is more of an infiltrator, slowly weaving its many-faceted web of sensuousness. Give it time to breathe and work its spell on you. You may well find it quite irresistible.

What to wear it with, where and when

Trésor adores all the soft shades of all colours, especially peach, apricot, plum, mandarin, rose, dusky pink, powder blue, lilac, dove, celadon, cream and tobacco. It's quite successful with black, but isn't much chop with white. The fabrics it loves are velvet, satin, brocade, fine wool, georgette and organza. Everything must have a genteel refinement about it, which doesn't mean you have to look like a dowager. In fact, quite young women are lovely wearing it, as are women of most ages. Not for the out-doors, but suitable for almost anything else, **Trésor** is the perfume to wear when you want to cut a quiet dash.

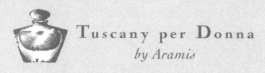

Tuscany per Donna
by Aramis

PRONUNCIATION: TUS-kan-ee pear DONN-uh ARRA-miss

*Y*ou might be forgiven for thinking that someone wearing **Tuscany per Donna** was actually wearing Guerlain's **Samsara**. At my first smell of this quite exhilarating perfume I must admit to doing a double-take – that is, until the air settled and I realised it was quite different from what was probably its inspiration.

This is not to say it isn't a very charming and ingratiatingly feminine perfume. Indeed, **Tuscany per Donna** is rich and vibrant, with a surprising subtlety and substance.

One could go on at length about its supposed tribute to the scented hills of Tuscany and its analogy to the so-called New Renaissance Woman, who is saddled with the job of straddling the old and the new with elegant assurance. More to the point is its intriguing and complex composition – a lovely *mélange* of sun-warmed flowers and sparkling citrus notes with flashes of spice. To me it smells overwhelmingly of jasmine and sandalwood, accompanied by rose, lily of the valley, hyacinth and ylang ylang. This gives it a rich tapestry, a velvety and soft opulence. Effervescent bursts of grapefruit and mandarin add a warm deliciousness that's given a slight edge with cypress oil, then mellow sandalwood adds its sophisticated, quiet strength and a small explosion of vanilla and amber lights it all with a show of distant fireworks, further releasing musk and frankincense.

The whole perfume does indeed evoke a Tuscan impression of terracotta sunsets, peach-blush mornings and bright days ablaze with hazy wildflowers. Its pastoral freshness is its strength, and its sweetness the secret of its charm.

What to wear it with, where and when

Tuscany per Donna requires romantic and totally feminine clothes in soft colours and fine, supple fabrics. It's a perfume that tends to float and insinuate rather than stride with overconfidence. Age doesn't matter to it very much, but the woman who suits it best is warm and charming, witty but unpretentious. She loves life and lives it to the full, as relaxed at a big gathering as she is entertaining quietly at home. Most of all, she is romantic, but not a sentimentalist – in fact, although she likes receiving flowers, she'd rather choose her own.

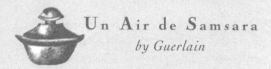

Un Air de Samsara
by Guerlain

Guerlain usually sets trends, not follows them, so it's surprising that this perfumer only recently entered the new arena of lighter, fresher, evergreen (meaning to be worn all year round) fragrances. Even more surprising is that it's done what Dior and Givenchy did with two of their classics, **Poison** and **L'interdit** – spinning off versions of them that are not merely *eaux de toilette* or *eaux de parfum*, but fragrances in their own right. After all, both **Tendre Poison** and **Fleur d'interdit** are very different formulations from their mentors.

So here we have **un Air de Samsara**, which is *almost* like the original **Samsara** in its overall statement, but quite individual at the same time. Beautiful and evocative, fresh and exhilarating, melodic and joyous, **un Air de Samsara** adds a few notes not emphatically prevalent in the mother perfume, becoming very much its own entity.

Un Air de Samsara's first exultant notes are citrus and mint, which gives it the piquancy of a pure *cologne*. Then, just as your senses are adjusting to this unexpected zing, lovely green notes give the middle notes their say with an enchanting trio of jasmine, narcissus and iris. The jasmine is uppermost to keep the essential **Samsara** theme pulsating warmly, but the coup is, of course, the same creamy, dreamy Mysore sandalwood used so lavishly in the original, but here used more sparingly. This gives **un Air de Samsara** the same haunting quality of **Samsara** but with a less sultry intensity. Rather than being in the shadow of **Samsara**, it lives its own light-headed, joyous life.

What to wear it with, where and when

Though designed to be worn all year round, I think its charms are much more obvious in the warmer seasons, particularly during midsummer idylls. It's the sort of smell that actually inspires confidence, so if you're a touch shy it will bolster you beautifully. **Un Air de Samsara** loves delicate colours, especially pastels and light metallics. Don't go overboard with the wardrobe – that's its mother's territory! Simple, youngish clothes, casual or slightly dressed-up, are best. Women from sixteen to sixty can wear it with ease and feel relaxed and self-assured in it.

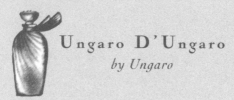

Ungaro D'Ungaro
by Ungaro

PRONUNCIATION: oon-GAR-o doon-GAR-o

As you'd expect, Ungaro's signature perfume is as startling and as sensual as his clothes. Anyone familiar with his unique niche in *couture* will know he's the doyen of the drape, the swathe and the pleat. Everything he touches is transformed into the near-fantastic in an unnerving juxtaposition of contrasting and clashing colours, fabrics and prints. The results are unfailingly individual and daringly successful.

It's this technique, this dash and bravura, that he carries over so well into his perfumes, and **Ungaro D'Ungaro** is no exception. It is dynamic, definite and exotic. So, if it comes on as a shock when first you try it, stay with it until the volatility unfurls into waves of mysterious depths.

Woods are a vital part of its intricate composition, especially sandalwood, which is added to the creamy caramel lushness of tonka bean and the spiciness of cardamom pods. This eastern treasure trove then meets the Middle East and the Mediterranean with heady orange blossom and Turkish roses, Florentine iris and Grasse jasmine. The harmonies are unusual, flung together in a passionate accord that strikes sudden sparks while dark notes throb sensuously underneath.

Ungaro D'Ungaro's powers of outright seduction are formidable, just like its majestic bottle shaped as a female and draped in poison blue, topped with a gleaming emerald and tied with vivid fuchsia ribbons. *Très formidable et très, très Ungaro!*

What to wear it with, where and when

Only the most sophisticated clothes need apply! This perfume's drama must be complemented and extended with well-cut clothes, spectacularly coloured or in straight black. No pastels, no in-betweens – all must be vivid and unequivocal, like the woman who can wear **Ungaro D'Ungaro** with style. She certainly won't be young or naive; rather, she'll be poised and self-assured. She's much more at home with lavish occasions than going on a picnic, and loves nothing more than making a big entrance and becoming the centre of attention. She also knows it is a perfume that totally ignores seasons and the time of day – just as she does.

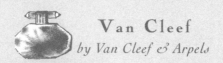

Van Cleef
by Van Cleef & Arpels

One look at the bottle, a many-faceted, sparkling jewel with an imposing gold stopper, and you know you're in the big league. **Van Cleef** is one of the most outrageously, unashamedly persuasive perfumes I know of. It is opulent, elaborate, extravagant, alluring and totally unavoidable – in the nicest possible way. Having the elitist credentials of one of the world's great jewellers, you know immediately that **Van Cleef** is all class!

It comes on strong, leading you into a whirl of what smells like tuberose but actually isn't. Its top notes are mainly bergamot and orange blossom, both very demonstrative and tenacious essences, backed with a deliciously vagrant and witty whiff of raspberry. This sends it off into a high-flying stratosphere, carrying with it a fabulously heady bouquet of roses and jasmine, vanilla from the Bourbon Islands, and that great stayer, tonka bean. Heady is the word as **Van Cleef** literally sweeps you away into exotic, sumptuous pleasures not quite of this world. There are no thoughts of intricate base notes – the perfume seems to fire of its own volition, and keeps firing for a long time. It's highly tenacious but never annoying.

Van Cleef is too self-assured and haughty to recognise competition. But it is so delicious it is irresistible! Subtlety is not in its vocabulary, though refinement is – like the jewellery house it represents so brilliantly. To wear it is to feel that same brilliant opulence.

What to wear it with, where and when

If you fancy yourself in an original Dior or a Saint Laurent, you'll most likely need **Van Cleef** to complete the drop-dead effect. This perfume is made for clothes of grand design and shattering effect. It can also descend the social scale to smart but dazzling cocktail dresses, zappy little suits and long swathes of chiffon or silk. It best makes its presence felt in jewel-like colours like emerald, sapphire, topaz, ruby and amethyst (anything pale and subtle is abhorrent to it). **Van Cleef** rises above all seasons and doesn't care if it's starred day or night, as long as it gets top billing. If you're on the prowl, on the town, or on a seriously seductive mission, don't leave home without it.

Vanderbilt
by Gloria Vanderbilt

*A*merica's fabled 'poor little rich girl', or 'Little Gloria' as she is often called, seems to have spent a good part of her life trying to swallow the silver spoon she was born with. As something of an individualist, her signature perfume is a testament to her emphatic style in the face of unfair criticism. It is both brave and stylish.

Vanderbilt is one of those like-it-or-loathe-it numbers. Personally, I think it's a very creditable perfume. It is highly complex, beautifully balanced and richly wooded. If that makes it sound like a wine, then the analogy fits – **Vanderbilt** has a lot in common with a good cabernet sauvignon.

A good deal more sophisticated and aloof than most of its American-born sisters, it is soft, subtle and rounded. The perfume is so cleverly constructed that its journey from top to middle through to base notes is gradual and pleasant – like a leisurely trip through the countryside, terminating at dusk at a pretty destination. There's not one bump on the way, not a jolt, no screeching of brakes. **Vanderbilt** is totally serene and unflappable.

It starts with a top note of heady flowers – orange blossom, tuberose and jasmine. Then comes the sharp addition of chypre to give a resinous, greeny ambience to the central notes, along with a beautiful selection of woods and dashes of bittersweet coriander that lead into an oriental panoply of vanilla and chocolaty Siamese benzoin. Glorious as each of these ingredients may sound in isolation, you'd be hard-pressed to separate one scent from another. The only thing that stands out clearly is the unique smell of **Vanderbilt**!

What to wear it with, where and when

Anything that smacks of the civilised street-smart chic of New York fashion suits **Vanderbilt**. Its cool, businesslike poise is great for refined occasions like the opera or ballet, where it revels in witty conversations during interval but genuinely concentrates on the artisitic content as well. Black, brown, navy, olive, taupe and amethyst suit its haunting woodiness – no pastels, thanks! Seasons don't ruffle its feathers and it's fine afternoon and evening. It's not for the very young, but it doesn't give a hoot if you're twenty-five or ninety-five – which is always comforting!

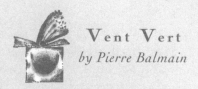

Vent Vert
by Pierre Balmain

PRONUNCIATION: varn VAIR
pee-AIR bal-MARN

*W*hat a joy to be able to include this very great and extremely lovely perfume! After enjoying quite some celebrity in the forties, **Vent Vert** seemed to fall out of fashion when the complex aldehydic florals and orientals took over the scene. It became extremely difficult to find and virtually vanished.

But the gods of perfume work in strange and devious ways for, lo and behold, **Vent Vert** suddenly reappeared. Of course, sometimes for things to remain the same things must change, and wouldn't you know it, **Vent Vert** is not *entirely* as we knew it. It doesn't have the same raw, uncompromising clout or indefinable sharpness as the original, but still bears a strong enough resemblance to its illustrious forebear. Although it's still hard to track down, it's a lovely discovery for those who've never heard of it before.

Vent Vert is as green and lush as grass, and as mesmerisingly tangy. It's the only perfume I know of that can evoke, even catapult you, clear into a calm and sunny summer's day in a flower-strewn field, and keep you hypnotised in its heady spell until the sun goes down on it with a whisper of breeze carrying it elsewhere. It does this by the surprising addition of a powdery note that clings as the green image fades.

Vent Vert is a delicious mystery. It's a glorious *mélange* of leaves and grasses, oakmoss and vetyver, bergamot and orange blossom, green rose and galbanum, sandalwood and fern, lily of the valley and jonquil, hyacinth and a fascinating edge of spiciness that might or might not be nutmeg. It's all part of the mystery. All I can say is, thank heavens it's come back to us on its delicious green breeze.

What to wear it with, where and when

Vent Vert's sharpness and achingly nostalgic beauty give it a lyrical presence day and night during the warmer months of the year. Naturally it was born for all the greens, from palest pistachio to darkest forest. It's also ravishing with yellow and stunning with white. Clothes must be unfussy, simple and youthful. It's a knockout, for instance, with a white linen suit, a green scarf and a stylish straw hat. The very mature might find it a bit too sharp and astringent, but the young and young-mature revel in it, as do sophisticates with an unconventional streak. Remember, it's nostalgic rather than romantic, so wear it accordingly, especially outdoors.

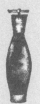

Vivid
by Liz Claiborne

Created as an antidote to the fresh and fruity, green and clean bunch of goody-goody perfumes that seemed to be choking the perfume market, Liz Claiborne designed **Vivid** to be the exact opposite – rich, vibrant and full-blown: vivid, I suppose you could say!

As a perfume it certainly doesn't hide its light under a bushel. It's a lovely, big, open and honest charmer that gathers together opulent full-scented flowers in a fabulous fantasia. The top notes come with a sudden rush of 'living' freesia, marigold, tangerine and a brilliant note of violet leaf. The freesia is so intense that when the soft floral centre of the bouquet emerges, it still gently persists. So the wonderful notes of jasmine, Bulgarian rose, peony, iris and a trio of gloriously unalike lilies – Amazon lily, lily of the valley, and tiger lily – join the pulsating freesia in a light-headed giddiness that's quite euphoric.

Vivid also has another little surprise up its sleeve. Creeping in under the base notes of sandalwood, vanilla and amber comes what Liz Claiborne calls 'the memory of the rare Tahitian tiare flower'. Tiare has a delicate but penetrating fragrance, somewhat resembling gardenia. Long after this perfume has settled on the skin, the notes that remain to haunt one are freesia, violet and the tiare flower.

Although definitely a romantic floral, **Vivid** is not subtle. For some women it may be slightly *too* vivid! But one thing to be said for this up-front perfume, it never overstays its welcome, having the grace to make a ladylike exit in a slow, haunting fade-out.

What to wear it with, where and when

The name solves it all for you. Anything vivid is bang-on, especially brilliant purple, green, red, orange and yellow. If you're into the blues make sure they're cobalt, electric or lapis lazuli. Metallics are great with it, but I'd leave the pastels, neutrals and greys well alone. Clothes should be romantic but not frilly, and fabrics should tend toward the opulent rather than the homespun. **Vivid** is definitely a party goer and loves to be out and about, but only after dark. It's fine in all seasons, particularly spring and summer, but make sure the youngsters don't get their hands on it – why should they steal your thunder?

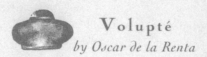

Volupté
by Oscar de la Renta

PRONUNCIATION: vol-OOP-tay

*H*aving been born, like Oscar, in the langorous tropics, I can be *simpatico* with the inspiration for this creation – all florid extravagance and flamboyance, with an uninhibited vividity of colour.

Volupté is an unashamed sensualist. Flooding the senses with an opulent cascade of flowers, it is pure luxuriousness. A lot of Yankee Gallicism in the guise of mystique has been heaped on the *raison d'être* for the name of this perfume, even going so far as to quote from Baudelaire's poem '*L'invitation du Voyage*' to describe its '*luxe, calme et volupté*'. But when all's said and done, the word itself simply translates as 'voluptuous' – no prizes for guessing that!

In de la Renta's hands, **Volupté** creates for itself an enitre world of beauty with its heady mix of freesia, jasmine and lots of violet. There's a beautiful dash of heliotrope, with its cherrywood enchantment, which then ushers in the lusciously ripe scents of melon and mandarin – a sensual path that leads to smouldering depths of musk, incense and patchouli tempered with soft murmurs of sandalwood. Thus the seduction completes itself, and **Volupté** emerges like a glittering butterfly – exquisite and utterly desirable.

This is a hugely rich scent that never once seems overblown. While it's not for the timid, it is supremely feminine and superbly poised. Invading and capturing the heart, it is impossible to deflect or forget. **Volupté** is a serious romantic.

What to wear it with, where and when

Purple and violet come to mind at the first whiff of **Volupté**, and to find the wearer in anything less dramatic is to know she hasn't understood its seriousness. It's a perfume that thrives on rich, vibrant colours – marigold, rose, amethyst, sapphire, cerulean, copper, jade – in fabrics such as silk, brocade, taffeta, satin, tulle and organza. It needs big dressing, like a huge hat or a startling turban over a sharp amethyst suit. As to age, nobody under twenty should touch it, while the over-fifties have probably run their voluptuous race and so don't need its sensuous flamboyance. **Volupté** is best in spring and summer, and if you're going to the tropics, take it along. It will really get those tom-toms throbbing!

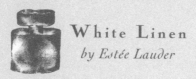

White Linen
by Estée Lauder

PRONUNCIATION: ESS-tay LOR-da

*T*his extremely successful darling of the Lauder fold epitomises the values of the homely family, the simple pleasures of clean living and the stripping away of overt opulence. With its goody-two-shoes scrubbed-clean image, it's a minor miracle **White Linen** has survived nearly two decades to become firmly entrenched in women's minds as a perfectly nice, socially acceptable and non-offending fragrance.

Why is it such a success? Probably because it's so undemanding and undemonstrative. It simply doesn't make waves. In fact, it barely manages a ripple, so well-mannered is its personality. But to call it dull or humdrum would be to do it an injustice. Despite the fact that most women who religiously wear it regard it as 'safe' (meaning comfortable, refreshing and refined), it is much more interesting and complex than that.

White Linen has an airy, breezy, almost breathless headiness, and although it's made from a richly scented floral bouquet, it doesn't actually smell very sweet at all. The presence of vetyver, that highly pungent Javanese grass-root, probably gives the game away, along with the soft citrus mellowness of mandarin. These together add a countrified air to the presence of Bulgarian rose and jasmine, along with strong infusions of lilac and lily of the valley. There's also a considerable whack of cedarwood and amber. Altogether these ingredients evoke a clear, breezy midsummer's day abuzz with bees and with birds twittering through fields of wildflowers. Romantic is too strong a word – perhaps 'captivating' is nearer the essence.

White Linen is honest and disarming, with a crisp clarity nicely softened at the edges – like a white raw linen dress trimmed with lots of broderie anglaise. Decent menfolk love it on decent womenfolk, and even kids like it on their mums!

What to wear it with, where and when

You shouldn't deviate too far from the fresh, crisp, just-laundered approach. Stick to white, cream, mushroom, grey, yellow, pale green and blue and all the pastels, patterned or plain. **White Linen** is definitely a daytime darling – wearing it at night requires a lot of effort, which may end up being inappropriate, especially when it has to compete with the big league. Let it hibernate in winter; spring and summer are its natural compatibles. Age is totally unimportant – you can give it as a gift to a grand-mother or granddaughter.

Wings
by Giorgio Beverly Hills

*I*f **Giorgio** and **Red** proved a bit much for the subtle tastes of some, the latest offering from this American perfumer wouldn't offend even your maiden aunt.

Wings is probably the first publicised 'committee' perfume ever made. Two thousand American and European men and women were targeted and questioned about their preferences in fragrances. From their responses, five perfumes were formulated. The testers were then sent these samples and asked to wear each of them for at least a day before making their evaluations. From their preferences a new perfume emerged – **Wings**.

Apart from its curious genesis, **Wings** has another unique attribute: it is one of the first perfumes to employ the process called 'living flower technology', where the smell of a live bloom is faithfully copied by chemistry. The finished product seems to have invented for itself not only a new category, but a whole new flower! **Wings**, being obviously a floral type at heart, doesn't smell like a lovely procession of flowers but like one single flower. A true holistic hybrid may be on the books!

Be all that as it may, **Wings** has a very pleasant smell. It's neither delicate nor sweet, and certainly not cloying or confronting. It begins with an ebullient burst of floral scents, which it maintains steadily for quite some time before it shifts slightly to the Orient with a soft woody background. In all, **Wings** is a welcome flutter from the overcrowded, raucously squawking perfume nest we've almost become immune to. It actually has restraint – a word I thought I'd never apply to anything from the venerable establishment on Rodeo Drive!

What to wear it with, where and when

Since **Wings** crosses most age-groups quite nimbly, keeping things simple, fresh, bright and exuberant is the best shot. It's principally an outdoorsy, fun-loving perfume rather than a heavily social one, so colours should be vibrant (plain or patterned), in cotton, denim, linen, light wool, rayon or silk. Clothes must be casual but well cut; the aim is to look crisp! Forget it in cold weather, and don't feature it at important meetings or occasions: **Wings** is for friendlier encounters. Think always of this perfume as if you're about to go on a long-awaited holiday – it loves to fly, naturally!

Y

by Yves Saint Laurent

PRONUNCIATION: EE (*not* WHY)

eve sarn lor-ON

*I*n 1964, two years after opening his own salon, Saint Laurent launched this, his first and most enduringly lovely perfume. Of all his perfumes, **Y** most reflects the underlying classicism and the astonishing originality of his clothes. It doesn't have the recklessness of **Rive Gauche** or the exotic orientalism of **Opium**, the hedonism of **Paris** or the dazzling lightness of **Champagne**. **Y** is more the perfumed summation of his style and richly inventive genius. Not only is it daring and beautiful, it is downright amazing!

Saint Laurent insisted on sheer perfection in every detail of this perfume. It must have immediate and unique appeal, it must be tenacious enough to remain popular, and it must be capable of becoming a classic. After all these years, all this has come to pass, even though a few years ago it took a virtual re-launch to put it firmly back in the public eye. Having 'rediscovered' it for myself recently, I found I had not forgotten its overt charm, its elegant allure.

Its initial sophistication comes from Bulgarian rose and Grasse jasmine with the soft, moist crush of oakmoss.

Oakmoss is a most unusual choice for such a dominant top note, but one which firmly sets **Y** on a very different avenue, strewn with a fetching bouquet of field flowers – narcissus, hyacinth and honeysuckle. This is given the luscious glow of peach, a breath of ylang ylang, the sharp tang of vetyver and a rush of green leaves. Warm, golden amber completes the brilliance. Everything ends, or rather dissolves, in a twilit, smoky smoulder . . . hauntingly beautiful and timeless.

What to wear it with, where and when

In the same way that nothing can be added or subtracted from a piece of Saint Laurent *couture*, so **Y** fuses with and complements the style of its wearer. It doesn't really matter if you don't possess a real Saint Laurent frock, it's the feeling that this perfume gives you as an individual that makes you feel so deliciously self-assured and elegantly poised. Wear it with red, black, white, grey and gold, either day or evening. **Y** transcends all seasons and temperatures.

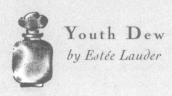

Youth Dew
by Estée Lauder

PRONUNCIATION: ESS-tay LOR-da

I still can't understand why this excellent perfume was given such a gauche name. But I guess, given its unique placing in the market way back in the fifties when it was launched, it's almost forgivable.

It started off as a concentrated bath oil that doubled as a 'skin perfume'. The concept was totally new, and **Youth Dew** hit the jackpot! Hitherto perfume had been preserved for formal or special occasions, but in light of its bathing properties, **Youth Dew** became a daily part of life and set the ball rolling with the idea of layering fragrance – from bath to after-bath, and finally using the perfume as the crowning glory.

Youth Dew is really more revolutionary than meets the eye. One would have expected such a blockbuster to be a floral bouquet bursting with rich and popular floral scents, but the amazing thing is that Lauder had the fearlessness to do it with an oriental. Although it's based on the usual Far Eastern line-up of intoxications, it has a unique, high-key top note of zesty citrus oils played against the sharp greenness of Geranium Bourbon from a Reunion Island. Once this is established (and it stays emphatically high for the duration of its life on your skin), the more serious sex-oriented ingredients come in for their wallop. There's sweet balsam and the chocolaty note of Vietnamese benzoin, the smouldering golden scent of labdanum (Spanish amber) and a caravan of roses, jasmine, carnation, clove, vanilla and musk, plus a good whiff of patchouli to really hold the cargo together for a long journey.

Naturally it follows that **Youth Dew** is anything but shy or subtle. Estée Lauder herself has described it as 'a very, very sexy modern fragrance'. So why not rediscover it and try your chances?

What to wear it with, where and when

Youth Dew goes all out for glamour and drama, so spectacular clothes in rich fabrics and colours are called for – plus a thick veneer of polish and sophistication to pull it all off. Don't overdo it or you'll quickly clear the room, but layer it on lightly from your bath onwards. It's a perfume for evenings only and is especially successful in the boudoir when worn with stunning black lingerie. It's certainly X-rated, so keep Granny well away from it in case she gets ideas beyond her capacity!

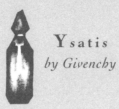

Ysatis
by Givenchy

Givenchy has probably been the most constantly elegant and unchanging of the Parisian *couturièrs*. He was always streets ahead of many of his flashier colleagues in style, mastery of cut, creation of line, and sheer panache!

Ysatis perfectly complements the summation of his *couture* artistry. It was created in 1984 and is the archetypal perfume in his collection. Givenchy wanted an encounter, a rendezvous between seductive feminine charm and its counterpart in perfume – something at once gentle, sophisticated and subtle. The creators of **Ysatis** gave him all that in spades! And they also gave him a totally new style of perfume, one that a lot of other perfumers would give their precious noses for. Instead of a three-movement symphony, clever **Ysatis** did it all in one! The myriad ingredients were so tightly bonded they didn't divide themselves into the traditional development of top, middle and base notes. So it's safe to say that what you smell first with **Ysatis** is virtually what you get and keep on getting until the perfume discreetly disappears.

Basically, it's a quartet of woods, flowers, fruits and spices bedded down with an almost dangerous liaison of earthy, sexy animal notes. Its woodiness comes from oakmoss, sandalwood and green galbanum; its floral chorus is led by Egyptian rose, jasmine, ylang ylang, iris and orange blossom; its spiciness is derived from essence of clove and vanilla; and its fruitiness comes from the tang of bergamot and mandarin. As if this alliance of Occident and Orient isn't seductive enough, it is then enveloped in a warm and clinging blanket of sultry Canadian beaver, Abyssinian civet, musk and amber – not so much a carnival of animals but a stampede of them!

In making **Ysatis**, Givenchy wanted to symbolise the mystery of Woman. With its civilised and tantalising allure, it achieves his goal with great elegance and finesse.

What to wear it with, where and when

The cultivated orientalism of **Ysatis** demands stylish, highly polished dressing, night and day. It loves rich, burnished colours, plus black and white, but is quite comfortable with the likes of lush moss-green or indigo. It suits all ages but the young, as long as the woman concerned is aware of its subtle powers, its warm urbanity, its elitist serenity. Autumn and winter are its shining seasons. **Ysatis** loves to be taken to where the lights are luminous, the company is witty and the prospects are dazzling!

A POTPOURRI

More perfumes A to Z

*T*he perfumes included in this section have consider-able worth in their individual ways. For a variety of reasons, however, be it lack of current popularity, the simplicity of their formulations, or pure prejudice and superstition on the part of perfume buyers, some of these perfumes have not enjoyed the same popularity and elevated status of many other perfumes, and some are a little difficult to purchase at times. Nevertheless I've felt they should be included, even if in more abbreviated form than those detailed before. Although they may be brief in description, these potpourri pleasures still have many individual charms and shouldn't be treated as barely worthwhile. Many of them are actually small masterpieces!

Carolina Herrera
by Carolina Herrera

PRONUNCIATION:

KARRO-lyna her-RARE-ruh

Once awarded the honour of 'The World's Most Elegant Woman', Carolina Herrera has successfully created a perfume that mirrors the style of her clothes – classical, romantic, clean. In these days of complex concoctions, its formula is almost austerely simple.

Carolina Herrera has been described as 'jasmine fireworks', and it does have an extraordinary amount of this spectacular scent. There's a fruity Spanish jasmine note, a romantic note of French jasmine and a lustier, stronger Indian jasmine essence that leaves you in no doubt about its sensuous intentions. Hot on the heels of this jasmine onslaught comes tuberose softened with a touch of sandalwood and fixed with amber and musk.

This is a very exuberant, exotic and sensuous perfume, bright to begin with but developing into something quite haunting and refined. Wear it with white and black and all the strong floral colours like buttercup, cornflower, rose pink and violet. Elegant suits and romantic gowns in the finest fabrics can be worn anywhere refined. **Carolina Herrera** is a perfume for the svelte, sophisticated woman to wear all year round.

Delicious
by Gale Hayman

ale Hayman's most infamous claim to fame is **Giorgio Beverly Hills**. Enough said. When testing her new perfume for the nineties woman, however, Ms Hayman got a universal response: 'It's smells delicious!' they all enthused. So **Delicious** was christened and let loose on the world. Though it smells very fruity, the top notes claim only one fruit – the lovely, insistent mandarin. This is accompanied by narcissus and mimosa for a light and sunny feel. The centre gets a little more serious, with a highly charged bouquet of rose, tuberose, jasmine, lily of the valley and ylang ylang.

Delicious is a perfume that goes out of its way to be 'thoroughly modern' via Rodeo Drive, but in truth it's really a nice, old-fashioned fragrance given a light-headed twist of freshness and outspokenness. To me it's sweetly enticing and voluptuous – a real softie that's all peachy and purring.

Wear it with pink, magenta, orange, yellow, amber and ginger, concentrating on the pretty and charming, not the flashy. The lighter naturals of linen, cotton, silk and chiffon suit its freshness and simplicity, as do all the seasons but winter. **Delicious** needs a woman who is bright, flirtatious, witty and subtly seductive, and probably in her late twenties to thirties. I think it might be a bit too sweet for the teenage disco set.

Duende

by J. Del Pozo

PRONUNCIATION: doo-END-dair
YAY-zuz del POTZ-o

*J*esus Del Pozo? Well might you ask! But not if you're a modern Spaniard. Del Pozo has been an acclaimed name in fashion circles for a number of years now. His signature perfume, **Duende**, which is Spanish for 'charm', is miles from the torrid, earthy and explosive smells we've come to associate with perfumes from that country. **Duende** is so cool it will take your breath away.

It starts with a lot of not-too-strident citrus notes with an 'aquatic' character, meaning they are reminiscent of the sea and sand. Then a mouth-watering melon essence emerges to bolster the outdoorsy freshness before a bouquet of jasmine and mimosa add their sweet sunniness. Smooth sandalwood and cedarwood are added, and finally a bunch of windswept thyme to permeate the entire accord.

Duende is the sort of fragrance you'd like to splash extravagantly all over you as if you'd just had a zingy turn in the surf. For day or evening, wear it elegantly cool and unfussy in all the sea colours, especially jade, sky blue, yellow and white, in summery fabrics like cotton, linen, chiffon and organdie. For the carefree, ingenuous and charming woman, **Duende** is as exuberant as a *zarzuela*, and just as satisfying.

Elysium
by Clarins

PRONUNCIATION: ell-EECE-ee-um

Clarins modestly describes this fragrance as 'Heaven on Earth', and it certainly does have ethereal qualities. In the first place, it's not particularly tenacious, being only an *eau de toilette concentrée*. Secondly, don't expect a thunderclap when you smell it. **Elysium** is more of a whiff of the fabled Elysian Fields – peaceful, tender, and very pretty.

Flowers dominate the accord. It combines freesia, lily of the valley, jasmine, *rose de Clarice*, osmanthus and the lovely linden blossom, adding fruity dashes of dewberry and papaya as a delicious counterpoint. This is then anointed with cedarwood and sandalwood, a hint of musk, and ginseng and ispaghul for their moisturising properties.

Elysium, true to its legendary name, conjures up broad vistas of cypress trees, babbling brooks, pan-flute music and dancing maidens. Not your particular cup of Paradise, maybe, but enough to satisfy the romantic sensibilities of most.

This is a perfume for celestial colours – pastels, white, silver and gold – and clothes that are filmy and diaphanous. Afternoon dalliances, baptisms and weddings are the places to take it, but make sure it's spring or summer, and keep splashing it on as it drifts away. **Elysium** is quite convincing, no matter what your age.

Escada
by Escada

PRONUNCIATION: ess-KAR-duh

Like the enormously successful German fashion empire after which it was named, **Escada** is vibrant, disarming, outspoken, international, and expensive. And although it has a highly complex composition, it comes across as a strongly modern synthesis of 'romantic' ingredients. The top, middle and bottom notes are so intertwined that all is fused successfully into one exultant shout that proves to be clear and tenacious.

Its flower notes are powerful collisions of sweet European hyacinth, heady Moroccan orange blossom and the eastern exotica of ylang ylang. This formidable trio is firmly bolstered with luscious peach and plum plus the citrus zest of bergamot. This is then orientalised with sandalwood and vanilla, and a final surprise of coconut to add a slightly tropical sweetness. The overall effect is vividly floral, a high-decibel pizzazz of calculated chic!

For the extroverted, witty and capricious woman, **Escada** should be worn to gossipy lunches with smart suits, tailored pants, *après-ski* wear or anything mannish. Red, gold, silver, orange, hot pink and saffron are its colours, in gaberdine, wool, polished cotton, silk, suede, taffeta, linen, lace and leather. Wear it all year round except in high summer.

The Floris Family
by Floris

PRONUNCIATION: FLOR-ris (as in 'Doris')

*P*urveyors of the finest English Flower Perfumes and Toiletries to the Court of St James since the year 1730. By Appointment to Her Majesty the Queen, Perfumers J. Floris Limited, London.' They don't come any more English! Or so you'd think. But Floris is, in fact, not an English name at all. It belonged to one Senor Juan Farmenias Floris from the Spanish island of Minorca. This young and determined perfumer transported himself to London at the start of the eighteenth century, married an English rose and set up shop in fashionable St James. His family has prospered ever since.

The beauty of the Floris range is that it's composed mainly of single-flower scents, so if you're the hearts-and-flowers type, why not build up a personal fragrance wardrobe of Floris favourites?

First up in the florals there's the classic **Ormonde**. This is a gloriously unusual marriage of wild things like green oakmoss, fern and soft musk with the more cultivated enticements of jasmine and rose. It has a lovely lingering presence, as if the fields and flowers were meeting in a lovers' tryst. Heaven for shady afternoons and genteel gatherings, it's especially kind to the woman of more mature years.

Florissa is a hedonistic, full-blown bouquet of highly sensuous flowers – English rose, lilac, jasmine, lily of the valley and iris – with a more sophisticated brigade of tropical Madagascan oils, woods and amber. A fascinating *mélange*, **Florissa** loves big floral prints and multi-coloured pastels, and thrives on debutantes emerging like brilliant butterflies.

Edwardian Bouquet is a slightly more formal, nostalgic charmer more suited to the debs' mums. It's anything but old-fashioned or musty, however, having a lovely, quiet pastoral tranquillity. It's luminous with wild hyacinth and night jasmine, and softly rounded with oriental echoes of sandalwood. Wear it all year round with tailored clothes and elegant evening wear.

Another of the feminine charmers is the majestic **Stephanotis**. The rapturous flower after which it is named is traditionally used in wedding bouquets. Here, Floris captures its precious essence and infuses it with notes of carnation, jasmine, petitgrain, coriander and, of course, bridal orange blossom. You don't have to go to the altar to wear it, and you'll find it ravishing when worn with white, pale blues, greens and mauves on spring and summer evenings.

Red Rose is an especially deep and rich rendition of the classic rose theme, but being made from the highly concentrated Attar of Roses and then blended with other rosy essences, it forms a rather regal stance. If you're the sentimental romanticist, you'll take it to your heart. It's perfect worn with unfussy, classically tailored clothes all year round, and blooms best on twilit evenings.

Moss Rose is much more veiled and mysterious than its sister. Its smoky, enigmatic depths are especially flattering on the more mature. Wear it with shadowed pink, rose, moss green, ruby and imperial purple to bring out its elusive but magnetic beauty.

Malmaison is my favourite of the Floris perfumes. A distillation of the aristocratic pink carnation of that name, it's one of the most imposing of the family and should be worn only by women with great style. It's a knockout with opulent evening dresses and devastating with black, white, gold, silver, cyclamen and all shades of pink and violet.

Wild Hyacinth is the Floris tribute to the ever-lovely English bluebell hyacinth, all foresty sweetness and shyness. It also has a green piquancy which tempers its heart-on-the-sleeve vulnerability with a cool and slightly wild freshness. Wonderful on the young, and perfect with pastels, it's terribly terribly English!

Rose Geranium is the rebel of the family. Mixing romantic rose notes with the pungency of Spanish geranium, it's very redolent of Spain – warm, spicy, sunny and passionate. Provided you have a touch of the non-conformist about you, age is immaterial to this perfume. Wear it with red, yellow, orange, emerald, hot pink, gold, white and black.

Lily of the Valley is at the opposite end of the spectrum, all dewy-eyed innocence and trembling delicacy. Its high-pitched, heart-aching sweetness is crowned with a soft green freshness. Perfect on the young in spring and summer when worn with simple and uncomplicated clothes.

Sandalwood blends the essence of this lovely, precious wood with sweet musk and creamy jasmine to emerge as a refined English impression of an oriental fantasy. To complement its slight aloofness, it should ideally be worn by mature women dressed in leather, velvet, wool and linen.

Limes, which is just as deliciously zesty on men as women, is a simple splash with strong, citrusy lime notes blended with the green breathiness of lime blossom to refine the slightly tart edges of the fruit. It's exhilarating without being astringent – perfect for spring and summer, and a natural with casual clothes in green, white and yellow.

Jasmine is the House triumph, faithfully capturing this heavenly (and often over-synthesised) flower in a distillation that is not overpoweringly strong or cloying. It is, of course, very rich and heady, but its lingering allure makes it perfect in warmer weather. It's particularly suitable for layering, from a luxurious bath to the final caress of toilet water.

No English garden is quite complete without **Lavender** – the quintessential variety with its nose-twitching, hay-like smell that's at once acerbic and warm. **Lavender** is not just for old ladies and lace, smelling enchantingly young and compelling on practically anyone at any time.

The youngest member of the family is **Zinnia**, named after a flower which doesn't have any scent of its own to speak of, but conjures up summer flowers bathed in Van Gogh sunlight. **Zinnia** is, in fact, a lilting blend of rose, iris and violet with a hint of spice. May it grow as gracefully as the rest of the 'By Appointment' Floris family. *Olé!*

Joop! Femme
by Joop

PRONUNCIATION: YOPE FAM

Wolfgang Joop, the successful German designer, does nothing by halves. When he decided to create a signature perfume, he introduced three simultaneously: **Femme** for women, **Homme** for men, and **Berlin** for both sexes. None of the three costs the earth.

Joop! Femme starts with a rose and jasmine alliance, but this is quickly overtaken by an extraordinary array of citrus notes. There's a powerful barrage of lemony bergamot and heady neroli, which comes from the unopened buds of the bittersweet Seville orange. Orange flowers are also present, and to add softness there's a hefty dash of hay-like coumarin and a soft infusion of sandalwood.

Joop! Femme is user-friendly and won't lead you into the deep waters of dangerous desires, or any other such *verboten* traps. It has enough niceness and sparkle, plus that little extra mischievousness, to loosen any inhibitions. For the office, a pop concert or a hearty restaurant, **Joop! Femme** is a good-natured perfume. If you're between twenty and forty, wear it all year round with casual but classy day wear, designer jeans and chunky fun jewellery. Colours are vibrant blues, reds and yellows, as well as white, gold and silver. But no neutrals, please – this is a German creation!

L'Aimant
by Coty

PRONUNCIATION: lay-MON
CO-tee

L'**Aimant**, or 'The Magnet', has been drawing people since 1927 when the great perfumer François Coty first began to experiment with aldehydes. He began with a great blooming bouquet of traditional roses and jasmine with a touch of jonquil and ripe peach placed over a sweet base of soft sandalwood, sharp vetyver and the animal warmth of synthetic civet. History has long since clouded over the rest of the ingredients, but the main thing is that **L'Aimant**, by virtue of its beautifully balanced formula, is full-throated, compelling and unmistakable.

Its fragrance has changed a little over the years, but it doesn't appear to have lost much of its heady beauty. While its presence today may be softer and sweeter, it still has the power of feminine seduction. I think it's an ideal choice for the young, and it remains a charming choice for the more mature woman who wants to remain attractive to men.

L'Aimant should be worn with anything bright and cheerful, especially strong primary colours. Smart casuals, flirtatious dresses, suits, pants and brief tops are simple enough to meet with its favour, and unsophisticated young gatherings are its place. Wear it all seasons with *joie de vivre*!

Maja
by Myrurgia

PRONUNCIATION: mah-HAH

my-RUR-ja

This Spanish perfume has always reminded me of
Bizet's passionate *Carmen*. Perhaps over the years my
nose's memory has left me with a stronger impression
of **Maja**'s power than it actually has. Or perhaps, like a lot
of perfumes, in order to survive the sales jungle it has had
its original formula altered somewhat. But whatever may
have happened, it's still a perfume to be reckoned with.

Maja's Catalonian clout comes from a brash bouquet
of *rose d'Orient*, jasmine, wild lavender and carnation overlaid with the darkly caramel smell of tonka bean essence. I
suspect there's also some pungent Spanish geranium lurking
in its depths, as well as plenty of patchouli, amber and
oakmoss to add sloe-eyed smoulder to the dazzling fiesta!

Like the flamenco **Maja** is seductive, like the bullring it
is magnetic, and like *España* itself it is grand, proud and
tempestuous. The woman who wears it must be all these
things. Her colours are red, scarlet, orange, gold, pink and,
above all, black. Clothes should be dramatic – big dance
dresses, capes, boleros, gaucho pants, tailored suits, black
lace lingerie. For any season but spring, **Maja** suits women
between twenty-five and forty, but definitely not blondes.

No. 4711
by Mülhens

*T*he original *eau de cologne*, and still going strong, so don't scoff at it! A complex mix of citrus and herbal ingredients including lemon, orange, bergamot, neroli, rosemary and lavender, **No. 4711**'s makers have stuck rigidly to this formula since before 1875, when its trademark was registered in Paris. Which brings us to its strange name and even stranger history.

In seventeenth-century Italy a young travelling salesman named Feminis distilled a theraputic formula called *aqua mirabilis*. He took his miracle water to the influential German town of Cologne, where it met with immense popularity. Before dying in 1763, Feminis left the precious formula to his son Giovanni Maria Farina. As luck would have it, a war between the French and Germans was in full swing, and French troops garrisoned in Cologne fell for the perfume in droves. The new heir to the *cologne*, one Wilhelm Mühlens, realising its latent popularity in France, quickly built a factory on the rue de Cailles. The street number was 4711.

No. 4711 is invaluable as a pick-me-up, especially in hot weather (keep it in the fridge), and is absolute magic when you're travelling, suiting all seasons, colours, clothes and occasions. It is extremely versatile, so please give it its due. Anything that's survived unchanged for some two-hundred-odd years must have something going for it!

Ô de Lancôme

by Lancôme

PRONUNCIATION: LARN-com

This wonderful *eau de toilette* has at last made a welcome return after an unexplained absence, so there's no excuse not to splash around in it with abandon!

Ô de Lancôme is a true original. Unlike its citrus-based competitors, it doesn't rely so much on the skin or the juice of the lemon but on the intense smell of the leaves. If you crush a lemon leaf in your hands you'll have an idea of the zingy tang of Ô. To soften some of the citric shock, a whiff of jasmine, some smooth green oakmoss and a base of sandalwood and vetyver are added. It lasts very well, fading with exactly the same lemon-leaf smell it begins with.

It's impossible to imagine getting through summer without it. One sniff and you'll be transported to the middle of a lemon grove under a clear blue Mediterranean sky, the smell of new-scythed hay in the next field, the gurgle of a creek gushing from a hillside spring and a passing waft of jasmine tantalising your nose. Bliss!

Ô de Lancôme is perfect with yellow, cream, white, green and any pastel except pink, and simple clothes in light fabrics like cotton, silk, georgette, linen, piqué. It's strictly for spring and summer, and especially good at *al fresco* gatherings. A word of advice – keep it hidden from *him*!

Ombre Rose
by Jean-Charles Brosseau

**PRONUNCIATION: ombrr ROSE
zjhon-sharl BROSSO**

a perfume more famous for its bottle than its availability, **Ombre Rose** is difficult to come to terms with, I suppose because its name conjures up an image that's altogether different from its scent.

Literally, **Ombre Rose** means shadowy rose-pink. Which is just as well, because the roses in it are very shadowy indeed! Its main components are woods (mainly Brazilian rosewood and sandalwood) and vanilla – a contrasting sweet and dry harmony with a common denominator of softness. Over this is arranged lots of Florentine iris, plus tropical ylang ylang and musk and a surprising glow of honey. The effect is disturbing, definite and quite enigmatic, like finding yourself in a dark forest after a downpour with pungent earthy smells and exotic flower scents all around you.

Wear **Ombre Rose** with anything shadowy, like moss rose, dusky pink or frosted grey. Clothes should be very sophisticated, either tailored or draped, with even a touch of fantasy. Save this perfume for intimate dinners, concerts and meaningful modern art exhibitions. For autumn and winter only, it suits the mature, the assured, the mysterious and the kinky. Make sure you're well over twenty-one.

Roma

by Laura Biagiotti

PRONUNCIATION: LOW (as in 'wow') -ruh bee-aj-ee-OTT-ee

This is the Anna Magnani, the Sophia Loren, the Fellini of perfumes. It is so quintessentially Roman you don't have to go there to feel you're slap-bang in the middle of it. It is the lustiest, most outspoken fire-bomb you'll ever wear and live to tell the tale!

Roma's lethal magic is cardamom. Together with the sharp bite of mint and the intense citrus tang of bergamot, you have something resembling the effect of dynamite. Then the sweet power of roses, jasmine, lily of the valley and carnation are added to give the centre of **Roma** a full-blown allure that's just short of tempestuous. The heavies come in last to underline the whole ravishment: vanilla, patchouli, oakmoss, ambergris, balsam and myrrh.

Roma is a tigress, a siren, a vamp. It loves to be ablaze in orange, red, pink, gold, copper and brown. As far as clothes are concerned, the bigger, tighter and more low-cut the better. This is a perfume that craves glitzy social occasions, and because of its formidable staying-power it glides happily on into the wee small hours. It's Adults Only territory, and although a bit strident for spring, doesn't give a hoot about seasons. But do keep it for evening only.

Sculpture
by Nikos Parfums

PRONUNCIATION: skulp-TOOR
NEE-koss pa-FOOM

Coming from the Greek-born, Paris-based designer of intimate apparel, Nikos Aspostolopulos, **Sculpture** is, as you'd expect, redolent of the Mediterranean – intensely exhilarating and sparkling. Its creator likens it to the Elixir of Life, no less!

Its immediate notes are the citrusy excitement of bergamot and verbena. Then comes the sensuality of Turkish rose and Italian jasmine and violet – very persuasive and quite pervasive without tipping the general idea over into sultriness. Underscoring all this is an overtly sensual alliance of vanilla, sandalwood and tonka bean. Finally there's a dash of Italian orris to give it a warm, sunlit glow.

Sculpture doesn't send out powerful vibrations like seductive bouzoukis strumming an insistent love song. It's much more low-key and romantic, sending out its quiet messages with a promise of amorous things to come. Aphrodite would be pleased!

It's best with blues, yellows and white, and shines in casual clothes as well as Greek goddess drifts of chiffon and silk. **Sculpture** is for the young to the mature woman. It's lovely in spring and summer, especially when the sun's out.

Tea Rose
by The Perfumer's Workshop

They don't come any rosier than this. **Tea Rose** is the most intensely concentrated and astonishingly faithful rose fragrance you're ever likely to smell in a bottle. Although it goes firmly against Coco Chanel's famous statement that 'no woman wants to smell like a rose-bed', **Tea Rose** certainly proved otherwise when it burst upon us fresh from America. Its success at first was enormous – in fact, it seemed as if every woman was turning herself into a walking, talking rose! The fervour has since died down a touch, but **Tea Rose** has survived.

I take my hat off to its makers. It's hard enough these days to find a single-flower scent that is thoroughly faithful to its source, but to find one that has the ability to capture the essence and evocation of the tea rose with stunning clarity is a minor miracle!

Some may find **Tea Rose** a little too rosy for their tastes. But if you damned-well want to smell like a rose garden, and to hell with Chanel, do be careful with its application; it's very tenacious and may offend sensitive noses. Wear it with red, pink, pastels, silver, white and cream in fine cotton, linen, chiffon, organza and silk. Day or night, filmy, floaty feminine numbers are its thing, and parties, picnics and dances its occasions. Naturally it's a perfume for spring and is happiest on the young.

Tendre Poison
by Christian Dior

PRONUNCIATION: TOND-ruh PWAH-son

Non! Non! It's nothing like the fire-eating **Poison**, so relax! In 1994 Dior decided to pour gentle oils over troubled waters with the launch of **Tendre Poison**. Though announced as a new interpretation of the same theme, **Tendre Poison** is in fact utterly different from its namesake, opting for a gentler, fresher, more youthful ambience. It's like sipping a champagne instead of downing a Black Russian.

Tendre Poison begins with top notes of green galbanum and mandarin followed by heady freesia and orange blossom. The final accord is provided by the beauty of rich sandalwood and the creamy sensuousness of vanilla.

This is a fragrance of considerable beauty, but it is a youthful beauty with a devil-may-care impertinence – quite captivating and anything but seductive like its big sister.

Tendre Poison was made for every opalescent shade your heart desires. It's best in feminine but not necessarily frilly clothes, and handles day or evening wear with a gentle poise. It's charming in fine cotton, chiffon, lace and crêpe de Chine. A touch too tender for winter, it's wonderful in spring and summer, especially on the young and the young at heart.

True Love

by *Elizabeth Arden*

*I*f you remember Bing Crosby crooning sweetly to Grace Kelly in *High Society*, you'll no doubt recall that the song was 'True Love', a rather treacly ditty that went on to win an Oscar and feminine hearts everywhere. Now comes a fragrance that resurrects the Crosby–Kelly romance with a touch of nineties commonsense.

True Love is light, sweet and delicately floral, using two unusual ingredients to give a misty-eyed harmony. These are the lovely White Cloud Rose and the elusive but haunting lotus blossom. Accompanied by freesia, lily of the valley and a floral tangle of jasmine, iris and narcissus, they are the heart of the perfume. To consolidate this delicacy, a hint of sandalwood, musk and a bracing dash of vetyver make a subtle counterpoint. It's all quite charming and nostalgic.

This is a perfume to celebrate the attainment or remembrance of true love. As you'd expect, it suits every shade of pink, blue and mauve you can lay your hands on. Clothes should be very simple or very frilly, whatever you like, but nothing dramatic or remotely controversial. Great for blushing brides, **True Love** is a summer and spring perfume for any woman between eighteen and eighty, as long as she's a true romantic. It loves afternoon teas, intimate dinners, weddings, and is not averse to a sunset cruise with a new-age Bing at the helm.

Tweed
by Yardley

or as long as I remember, poor old **Tweed** has had an unfortunate image as a perfume for women who don't wear perfume. It is also indelibly associated with ageing aunts and musty grandmothers. All of which is absolute bunkum: **Tweed** is a totally charming perfume, and far from shy.

It makes its presence felt immediately with a strong rush of flowers backed by equally strong spices and woods. There's jasmine and carnation with zesty citrus oils and what smells to me like a hint of violet – the leaves as well as the flowers, and probably even the roots! This all comes together for a delicious wildness that's softened with sandalwood and given a sensuous persistence with musk.

Why it's called **Tweed** I have no idea. It doesn't remind me at all of the fabric, nor even particularly of Scotland. It's quite a stylish perfume, so don't treat it as a safe standby to be worn only with twin-set and pearls over high tea, please!

Suiting all seasons, but especially autumn and winter, **Tweed** is best with warm and earthy tones, plus black, white, cream and grey. For home entertaining, flower shows, lunches and shopping, it is the domain of the self-assured, charming and witty woman, whether she's a young mum or a doting grandma. It's a bit too serious for teenagers.

Venezia
by Laura Biagiotti

PRONUNCIATION: ven-ETZ-ee-uh

LOW (as in 'wow') -ruh bee-aj-ee-OTT-ee

This sister perfume to the more explosive **Roma** is not much less volatile in its initial impact. As befits its name, it is elegantly ethereal, exuding a tranquillity like early-morning mist on a Venice canal.

Venezia begins its swan-like journey with amazingly exotic notes of mango and blackcurrant bud with a hint of rich plum. Soon, though, it is suitably garlanded with a wonderful bouquet of jasmine, freesia, rose, iris, ylang ylang and the enigmatically sweet little wong-shi flower, a fragrance which in medieval times was used as an aphrodisiac by the romantic Venetians. The base notes come in last and are anything but shy – Indian mango, cedar, and those two sultry seductresses, vanilla and musk.

I like **Venezia** for its evocation of an enigmatic place. It insinuates, fascinates, excites and stays long in the memory, just as gliding down the Grand Canal in a gondola does. For the sophisticated and naturally elegant woman, it's a perfume to be worn from late afternoon to evening in dreamy, romantic clothes that float on the breeze. Colours should not be dark or dramatic, but pale and mysterious. It's best in spring and summer and quite charming in autumn.

A SCENTED STAR SEARCH

The perfumed zodiac

I firmly believe that certain fragrances or types of fragrances are more suited to some people than others. So if you either believe, are fascinated or merely amused by the powers of astrology to define each of us by our characteristics and our philosophies, there's no reason why it can't give indications as to the correct choice of perfumes we would like to think complement our psyches.

My aim is to outline each star sign's overriding or dominant fancies and foibles, as well as uncover some of the idiosyncracies each sign hides under its hat and apply these to specific perfumes. By doing this we can sniff out which smells you respond to emotionally, which ones you can wear with comfortable assurance and which ones to avoid. It's all in good fun!

Aries

You must be so used to having your foot in your mouth you need a pretty strong battery of perfumes to camouflage your embarrassment. Being a loud person (especially when you laugh at someone else's blunder) you need outspoken perfumes that make definite statements. Subtlety means nothing to you, so go straight for the bottle of **Giorgio Beverly Hills** or Gianfranco Ferre's explosive **Ferre**. Giorgio's other powerbroker, **Red**, is right up your alley too, as is Lauder's brooding sex-bomb **Youth Dew**. But underneath all this bravado you're really a child at heart and therefore adore pretty things, so when you've quite exhausted yourself and need to recharge those batteries, do yourself (and everyone else) a favour and fall into the liquid embrace of Grès's charming **Cabochard** or Dior's spicy **Miss Dior**. Even a dash of Lauder's serene **White Linen**, Saint Laurent's chic **Rive Gauche** or Lancôme's dreamlike **Pôeme** will help. Then, when you've had enough of peace and quiet, you can go out into the world and cause well-meaning havoc all over again. At least you'll smell nice.

Taurus

Okay, so you're sophisticated enough to negotiate a china shop without demolishing it, but that's only on a *good* day! If you're having a stinker of a one it's probably your fault, even though you'd be the last to admit it. So calm down, stop snorting rage and have a squirt of Rochas's delicious **Femme** or its lighter-intentioned **Deci Dela**. With their warm, witty elegance and charm, either of these ought to bring you back to the delights of the earth. Or you could try a touch of Roman warmth and welcome with **Fendi** or Biagiotti's **Roma**. In any case, you'll soon be back grazing away in your peaceful, electric-fenced paddock. This will give you time to ruminate on romance, the thing you really crave, and nothing will dish it up to you more tastefully than Givenchy's ardent **Amarige** or even a nostalgic whiff of Worth's **Je Reviens**. Other savage-breast soothers are Givenchy's smooth and seductive **Ysatis**, Chanel's earthy **No. 19** and the fruity orientalism of Chopard's **Casmir**. But if you must make a grand entrance into the bullring, have a lash at Armani's wondrous **Gio**, Paloma Picasso's voluptuous **Mon Parfum** or even Fendi's oriental **Asja**. Frankly, though, you'd be better off peacefully chewing your cud on Perfumer's Workshop **Tea Rose**, Lancôme's pacifying **Trésor** or even the ever-reliable cool charms of **No. 4711**. Your moo will be much more persuasive and you might even end up being seduced instead of seducing!

Gemini

As beautiful, busy and demented as a butterfly, anyone would think the bubbles in your glass would never go flat, mainly because you saturate yourself in the camouflage of flashy, effervescent perfumes like **Moschino** and **Oscar de la Renta** or Saint Laurent's dazzling **Champagne**. And fair enough! They smell great on you. So does the eternal **Joy** by Patou. But, let's face it, you are many-faceted (some might even suggest schizophrenic!) and there are other less capricious perfumes that may soothe the dark side of your soul. Perhaps you should learn to give in to the charms of Aramis's **Tuscany per Donna** or **Carolina Herrera**, or even the sweet libations of Dior's **Tendre Poison**, though personally I think your brand of charm is better suited to the not-too-dizzy heights of Ungaro's **Senso** or the mischievous flirtations of Versace's **Versus Donna**. In any case, butterfly or not, your wings usually get singed, so stay away from the big flames and settle for something less dangerous like Grès's younger-than-springtime **Cabotine** or the gently incandescent **Bvlgari**. You might even convince some people you're actually innocent and relatively sane!

Cancer

You're probably sick to death of the smell of baked dinners, endless flower arranging classes and anything to do with babies except cuddles. Why do you insist on being the happy little homemaker and Mother Courage all in one? If you had any sense you'd hire a babysitter and a stretch limo and drag your other half kicking and screaming out into the wilds of the night, having doused yourself in Saint Laurent's half-wicked **Opium** or the super-elegant **Kenzo**. Throw away all those mimsy toilet waters and rose perfumes and lose yourself in the wilder shores of **Boucheron** or the perverse pleasures of **Jean-Paul Gaultier**. You could even go the whole hog with Boucheron's **Jaipur** or the tropical **Fidji**. If you're still a bit daunted by the big guns, at least give yourself half a chance with Dior's ravishing **Diorissimo** or Guerlain's **Jardins de Bagatelle**, but I really think you're more suited to the intimate whisperings of Guerlain's **Chamade** and Saint Laurent's drop-dead **Y**. And when you've lullabied the last baby to sleep and put out the cat, keep your husband in with a devastating dash of **Romeo di Romeo Gigli**. He'll never buy you another bunch of boring old daisies again!

Leo

As a good Leo you have learned the laws of the concrete jungle and can brush up quite spiffingly for occasions. You'll polish your claws, comb your mane and be generally civilised, especially wearing something like Chanel's **Coco** or Lauder's **Knowing**. The latter might have been created specifically for you, since you are the know-all of the zodiac. Fortunately, lionesses take terrific pride in thinking they are the most sophisticated of all beings, and this means you can wear such haughty numbers as Givenchy's **Ysatis** and Hermés's **Calèche** with great aplomb. Actually, you'd be smarter if you considered down-playing the game a little with the unpredictable nuances of **Dolce & Gabbana** or Chanel's scintillating **Cristalle**. You tend, however, to think you can get away with the voluptuousness of **Shalimar**, which is a bit of a laugh because you're far too impatient for seduction; it's straight for the jugular with you! But if you're out for the kill there's no need for overkill, and you may find the cool sparkle of Saint Laurent's **Champagne** or Cartier's **Panthère** more suited to prowling than the usual block-busters you tend to parade around in. You may be an indefatigible fighter, but actually you're a softie underneath and will usually wilt under the spell of Patou's **Sublime** or a shot of **Gio** by Armani. Both are very golden perfumes which will suit your colouring and generosity and, who knows, they might even convince you to stop roaring and wander over to a shady tree for a nice long snooze.

Virgo

You criticise yourself so much you think it gives you the right to criticise others too, and are always the first to tut-tut any behaviour that doesn't comply with your stringent standards. The same applies to the way you choose a perfume. You nearly go bonkers trying to find the ideal one and are more than likely to be found wearing perfumes that are either too young for your years or too grand for your own self-effacing modesty. The one thing you have in your favour, though, is good taste, so a ritzy and elegant perfume like **Boucheron** or **Ungaro d'Ungaro** will satisfy your ego perfectly. Of course, the real truth about Virgoans is that underneath all that schoolteacher primness they are hopelessly romantic fools. If this is true for you then you're a sitting duck for Kenzo's charming **Parfum d'été**, the spring splendour of **Gianfranco Ferre**, Guerlain's tranquil **Mitsouko** or the enigmatic **L'Heure Bleue**. The sweetness of **Jean-Paul Gaultier** and the soothing libations of Shiseido's **Feminité du Bois** are good ideas, and I've yet to come across a Virgo who doesn't go weak at the knees over **Romeo di Romeo Gigli**. But I guess you'll go on feeling guilty about actually enjoying yourself, so to help your self-flagellation along I suggest a good lash at something really over the top, like Lauder's **Cinnabar** or **Gianni Versace**, or even the ritz of **Van Cleef**. Anything to cheer you up!

Libra

They don't come any vainer than you, nor more romantically nomadic! Without a mirror you're dead and without someone to seduce you are inclined to morbidity and sullenness. Of course, you don't see it that way. Unfaithful and fickle? Never! You're too level-headed and fair-minded for that. But you're convinced your love makes the world go around, and since you are the very centre of it, keeping peace with everyone is your way of telling the world you're simply the best! That's exactly why the sweeter and mock-innocent perfumes suit you best, like **Cabotine**, **Dolce & Gabbana**, **Tuscany per Donna** and Saint Laurent's rosy **Paris**. But when more seductive love potions are required for your undermining tactics, Lauder's **Estée** and Givenchy's **Amarige** are weapons without peer. And since women born under this sign are almost always pretty, what better than Dior's **Miss Dior**, Guerlain's **Jardins de Bagatelle** or Rochas's **Tocade** to complement your purring charms? But the best choice of all I think are the intimacies of **Carolina Herrera** or **Oscar de la Renta**, and Guerlain's matchless feminine troublemaker, **Chamade**.

Scorpio

Upstage you? Impossible! And unwise as well, knowing the Scorpion's appetite for deadly revenge. Actually, as a Scorpio you are more likely to upstage yourself, going way over the top and out of sight with no one bothering to tell you so! But as you swan imperiously through the hoi polloi, you do at least do it with panache. You're are so self-assured and haughty you naturally gravitate to perfumes that are unfailingly right for you, loving the drama and passion of such sirens as Dior's **Poison** and its less intense sister, **Tendre Poison**. You adore Guerlain's seductive **Shalimar** and Lancôme's mysterious **Magie Noire** and revel in the earthy lustiness of Paloma Picasso's **Mon Parfum**. Long ago you discovered that Desprez's **Bal à Versailles** could be a deadly weapon. As a matter of fact, Lucrezia Borgia has nothing on you. Even the summery charms of **Jardins de Bagatelle** and Lancôme's **Ô de Lancôme** take on a sinister sensuality when you wear them. You'll do anything to match the power of your self-confessed sexuality with a perfume of similar leanings, and powerhouses like Channel's **Coco**, Dior's **Dioressence**, Saint Laurent's **Opium** and even Calvin Klein's vampish **Obsession** are grist to your ever-churning mills. Though infamous for making a grand entrance, you're no match for the splendour of **Bvlgari** or Cartier's **Must**, both of which are so refined and elegant they could even manage to convince others that you have good taste!

Sagittarius

Hockey one, hockey two ... oops! Sorry old chum, didn't mean to break your leg!' You are such a good sport you tend to kill with kindness, so hearty, clean-minded and jolly you make people want to throw up — not that you'd ever notice: sensitivity is not one of your better points. Poor Sagittarius — loved but pitied, particularly for your total lack of good taste, which extends to perfume. You *will* insist on wearing the pretties, or the sexy heavies which are way out of your league. I suggest you build up a locker of fresh, uncomplicated and undemanding perfumes to suit your simplistic temperament. Throw out that **Tabu** and that **Giorgio** and try the subtler charms of Chanel's **No. 19**, Ricci's **Deci Dela** or the outright freshness of **Ô de Lancôme**. And if you're absolutely determined to be ladylike, then forget **Joy** (too feminine by half for you!) and go for Lauder's **Private Collection** or Worth's **Je Reviens**. The very best choices for you are thoroughbreds like Guerlain's **Jicky** and Lauder's **White Linen**. You can't go too far off the track with Saint Laurent's witty **Rive Gauche** or Dior's ozonic **Dune** either. And if you're convinced you need a touch of glamour, don't go for the bottle of **Shalimar** but opt for the warmth of **Fendi** or Ralph Lauren's **Safari**. You'll never play hockey again.

Capricorn

Climb every mountain, ford every stream, trample every person . . . It's a tough old life for you poor misunderstood goats, forever searching for a new summit to conquer, not because it's the tops but because *you* are! You're not just any old goat, you're highly bred, sure-footed, devastatingly charming and – let's face it – just about perfect! And so humble too! It was for you that Giorgio Beverly Hills painted the town **Red** and Saint Laurent faced the wrath of militant grapies just to pour your **Champagne**. Even Chanel must have had you in mind when she put super-ambitious aldehydes in **No. 5**. On a lesser but similar scale, you are just dandy in **Vanderbilt** and Lauder's **Youth Dew**, but please stay away from **L'Air du Temps** and go for Paco Rabanne's more flinty **Calandre** as a mark of respect. You might have a certain hard-edged femininity, but flowers on the breeze are not your scene. Deep down where it really counts, however, you are at your calculating, ambitious best in Ungaro's devious **Diva** and Gianfranco Ferre's drop-dead **Ferre**, and the ultimate achievement, Van Cleef & Arpels's **First**. They help when making earth-shattering decisions from the giddy heights of your towering stilettos and unassailable shoulderpads.

Aquarius

Heaven help you, you are the do-gooder of the zodiac – the hail-fellow-well-met type who others would dearly love to avoid! But as an Aquarian you give them no chance, tracking them like an over-friendly labrador. People know you mean well, but it all becomes a trifle sickening after a while. That's why you should always avoid perfumes of sweetness and light and go for the more calming, relaxing numbers like Estée Lauder's pretty **Pleasures**, Calvin Klein's **Escape** and Issey Mayake's pure and simple **L'Eau D'Issey**. If you have to dress up (and God knows you're no fashion-plate!), classics like Lanvin's flattering **Arpège**, Rochas's refined **Femme** or Hermés's slyly innocent **Calèche** are nice antidotes to your cloying altruism. Even the extravagance of Patou's **Sublime** or **Boucheron** might give you a more ladylike demeanour. Despite the Aquarian claim to being deep thinkers, you need more than a touch of chic to counteract your basic depressiveness. So when the real blues hit, take a shot of zingy, zippy Guerlain **Jicky** or the cool serenity of Kenzo's **Parfum d'été**. You'll have the bluebird of happiness ready to take off right up someone's nose in no time!

A Scented Star Search

Pisceans are labelled with just about everything, good or bad. Sensitive? Complex? Intuitive? Perhaps, but you are not *always* the pretty little periwinkle of the sea: sometimes you are an all-consuming piranha! You are the sort of person who leads a life other people envy – all dreams, drink, drugs and dangerous liaisons. But then, you are a terrible liar (you call it 'romancing') and cannot be trusted. Being a water sign it is ironic that you are terrified of the sea. Terra firma is where you'd rather be, and this accounts for your gravitation towards the green perfumes. You are at your happiest and floatiest in Balmain's **Vent Vert**, Guerlain's **Mitsouko**, Kenzo's **Parfum d'été** and Lancôme's lemon-leafy **Ô de Lancôme**. Keep well-stocked in extravagances like Guerlain's mystical **Samsara**, Desprèz's snobby **Bal à Versailles** and Cartier's ritzy **Must**, or if your budget doesn't run to that, assuage yourself with Armani's wonderful **Gio** or Lancôme's mysterious **Magie Noire**, or the beautiful **Gianfranco Ferre**. Being a Piscean, you are unmatched when it comes to making a big splash, so be sure you make your entrance in something as room-stopping as Paloma Picasso's **Mon Parfum**, Guerlain's **L'Heure Bleue** or Christian Dior's **Dune**. You just adore swamping the competition, even if it means drowning everyone else in the process!

INDEX OF PERFUMES

The Book of Perfumes